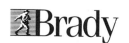

HAZARDOUS MATERIALS EXPOSURE

CONTINUING EDUCATION SERIES
Richard L. Judd, Ph.D., Series Editor

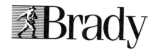

HAZARDOUS MATERIALS EXPOSURE

EMERGENCY RESPONSE AND PATIENT CARE

Jonathan Borak, M.D.

Michael Callan

William Abbott

With Contributions by:

Larry M. Starr, Ph.D.
Thomas McCarthy, EMT-P

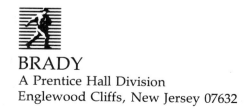

BRADY
A Prentice Hall Division
Englewood Cliffs, New Jersey 07632

Library of Congress Cataloging-in-Publication Data
Borak, Jonathan, 1946–
    Hazardous materials exposure : emergency response and patient care
/ Jonathan Borak, Michael Callan, William Abbott, with contributions
by Larry M. Starr, Thomas McCarthy.
        p.   cm.
    ISBN 0-89303-722-2 (pbk.)
    1. Medical emergencies. 2. Hazardous substances—Safety measures.
3. Emergency Medical Services. I. Callan, Michael, 1949–
II. Abbott, William, 1949– . III. Title.
    [DNLM: 1. Environmental Exposure. 2. Hazardous Substances-
adverse effects.   WX 215 B726h]
    RC87.3.B67 1991
    362.1'8—dc20
    DNLM/DLC
    for Library of Congress   90–1307
                                                                          CIP

Editorial/production supervision and
    interior design: Adele M. Kupchik
Cover photo: Eugene Kimball
Cover design: Ben Santora
Manufacturing buyer: David Dickey

© 1991 by Prentice-Hall, Inc.
A Division of Simon & Schuster
Englewood Cliffs, New Jersey 07632

Printed in the United States of America

10 9 8 7 6 5 4 3

ISBN 0-89303-722-2

Prentice-Hall International (UK) Limited, *London*
Prentice-Hall of Australia Pty. Limited, *Sydney*
Prentice-Hall Canada Inc., *Toronto*
Prentice-Hall Hispanoamericana, S.A., *Mexico*
Prentice-Hall of India Private Limited, *New Delhi*
Prentice-Hall of Japan, Inc., *Tokyo*
Simon & Schuster Asia Pte. Ltd., *Singapore*
Editora Prentice-Hall do Brasil, Ltda., *Rio de Janeiro*

CONTENTS

FOREWORD

Anhydrous ammonia, bromine, chlorine trifluoride, dimethyl sulfate, ethylene oxide, fluorine, hydrochloric acid, methyl sulfate, nitrogen trioxide, oleum, phosgene, sulfuric anhydride, and tetranitromethane are but a few of the *4 billion tons* of hazardous materials carried by our transportation systems by air, surface, and water. The warnings **DANGEROUS, EXPLOSIVES, FLAMMABLE SOLID, OXIDIZER,** and **CORROSIVE** are some of the signs used on transport vehicles, tank cars, or tank trucks. They tell responders to hazardous materials incidents to approach the incident cautiously. It is likely that many first responders have limited knowledge of the materials or warnings listed.

These hazardous materials are everywhere; they are an omnipresent emergency waiting to happen. No community—no matter its size, shape, demography, or economic focus (industrial, agricultural, commercial, service, retail, or residential)—is immune from the potential disaster of a hazardous accident. All of the materials listed earlier require initial isolation from a spill or leak from a drum or small container ranging from 50 to 600 feet. Larger spills increase the initial isolation and evacuation up to 3 miles!

Although accident frequency involving these materials is low, when accidents occur emergency action by public safety agencies must be on an informed basis. The hazardous materials scene is one to which the adage "For fools rush in where angels fear to tread" often applies tragically in the death of emergency personnel. For example, three unsuspecting emergency rescuers died in Lancaster county, Pennsylvania, attempting to rescue a child from a cistern full of cut grass and six firefighters died in Kansas City, Missouri, from the explosion of ammonium nitrate.

Hazardous materials have been with humankind since its origin; however, in contemporary times a global community using advanced technology develops and has available for daily use thousands of materials. These materials have allowed all of us to benefit thousands of ways in our daily lives. In fact, it is difficult to envision the world, as we now know it, without them. Yet, in the emergency service sector, we live with another reality. That reality faces us with exposure to several harmful activities and events. In the hazardous materials accident, no second chance may be available if EMS personnel make a mistake in dealing with the material involved.

Several texts in the available literature treat the hazardous materials subject matter; these are primarily (and properly so) directed to firefighters and rescue personnel for appropriate reasons. Others deal with definitive care in the medical facility; some detail chemical identification and properties.

The principal authors, Dr. Jonathan Borak, Michael Callan, and William Abbott, with contributors Dr. Larry Starr and Thomas McCarthy have written a different text. *Hazardous Materials Exposure* is the first text devoted to the EMS sector and hazardous materials.

The work provides a pragmatic view of EMS and hazardous materials incidents and accidents. It examines in a thorough yet concise manner, an orientation to the extensive material involved in hazardous materials training and education. The authors, from extensive and path-breaking experience, offer a comprehensive approach to hazardous materials for the EMS community. Recognizing the various ambiguities of current practice involving EMS in hazardous materials management, the authors have developed a text that offers a sensible education and training program for EMS providers.

The text in nineteen chapters presents material including hazardous materials behaviors, recognition of hazardous materials, assessment, personal protective equipment, decontamination, and physiologic factors of inhalation, and concludes with a well-conceived unit on stress related to the hazardous materials accident. The authors have done their job well; the benefits of a text devoted to the significant role confronting the EMS provider in a hazardous materials incident is long overdue. This work makes a timely and urgently needed contribution to the EMS literature.

Richard L. Judd, PH.D., E.M.S.I., N.R.E.M.T.A.
Series Editor
Executive Dean and Professor of Emergency Medical Sciences
Central Connecticut State University
Allied Medical Staff New Britain General Hospital
New Britain, Connecticut

PREFACE

Hazardous materials and the dangers they pose have become the subject of increasing concern all over the world. The American public, reacting with growing awareness to the extraordinary harm that industrial chemical leaks can cause, has demanded higher levels of emergency preparedness for hazardous materials accidents. Many of those demands have recently been formalized in federal and state laws. Examples are the broad, sweeping requirements of the Superfund Amendments and Reauthorization Act of 1986 (SARA) and related regulations developed by the Environmental Protection Agency (EPA) and the Occupational Safety and Health Administration (OSHA).

One part of SARA is Title III, also known as the Emergency Preparedness and Community Right-to-Know Act, which requires that emergency response plans for hazardous materials accidents be developed in every community of the country. That legislation marks the first time that standardized hazardous materials preparedness has been required throughout the United States. Complying with those requirements will pose one of the greatest challenges ever faced by emergency responders and the response organizations for which they work.

One of the important goals of those new legal requirements is to enhance the skills and knowledge of emergency responders. To accomplish that, there are extensive training demands. These specific requirements are discussed later (see Appendix 5). The regulations will have a large impact on emergency medical services (EMS) and other emergency medical personnel. To date, both hospital and prehospital emergency personnel have generally received little training about the risks of hazardous materials or the care of exposure victims. Similarly, acute industrial toxicology receives little attention in the curriculum of most medical schools and physician training programs.

This book is addressed to EMS personnel and other first responders who provide emergency health care to persons exposed to hazardous materials releases. We hope that this work will contribute to both the medical knowledge and performance skills of its readers. First we present information that all responders should know about hazardous materials: how they cause harm, how they can be recognized, and how to protect oneself from them. Next we consider hands-on EMS response procedures for hazardous materials incidents. Then we describe the health effects that result from hazardous exposures.

Good procedural skills are important for emergency responders dealing with hazardous materials. We think it is more important, however, that emergency response personnel appreciate the great dangers that these substances can pose to rescuers. Accordingly, we repeatedly return in this book to statements that emphasize the need for emergency personnel to protect themselves. The themes of these concerns follow.

Hazardous materials are great equalizers.   They can injure anyone who gets in their way, regardless of background, training, or intentions. Everyone at a hazardous materials incident must show concern for the potential harm of the chemicals involved.

The responder is the most important person at the incident.   EMS and other emergency personnel must accept responsibility for protecting themselves. Emergency responders should not needlessly expose themselves to avoidable risks of hazardous contamination. Nothing is gained, and a good deal is lost when responders become victims.

The first few minutes are critical.   What emergency personnel do during the first few minutes at a hazardous materials incident can shape the rest of their lives. Before allowing themselves and their colleagues to become exposed to hazardous materials, responders must evaluate the incident, determine its dangers, and plan a response.

Many hazardous incidents appear at first like "ordinary" nontoxic emergencies. This is especially true of transportation accidents. EMS personnel who react without adequate forethought and care are at increased risk of being exposed to toxic substances that can lead to illness and disability.

Finally, we must all recognize that despite the dangers created by hazardous materials, their value to our way of life makes doing without them all but impossible. We must accept living with them and learn to react as effectively and safely as possible when they are involved in accidents. To that end, we hope this book is a useful contribution.

Jonathan Borak, M.D.
Michael Callan
William Abbott

ACKNOWLEDGMENTS

This book is the product of efforts made by many more people than just those whose names appear on the title page. I wish I could acknowledge them all. My special thanks go to the following: Karen Muth, my closest associate, whose enthusiasm and competence have held this project together on more than a few occasions; Pat Wales, an excellent librarian and generous friend; the late Dr. Carl Monroe, former medical director of Rohm and Haas, who had foresight, understanding, and concerns about the public health dangers of industrial chemicals; Dr. Richard A. Lippin, medical director of ARCO Chemical Company, whose humanism invests his wide-ranging interests from industrial toxicology to arts medicine and poetry; Darrell Mattheis, a constant source of sound advice and encouragement; my many colleagues in the emergency medical, EMS, and fire service communities who have inspired, supported, and reviewed segments of this book as well as our other training programs; Dr. Jacek Franaszek, president of the American College of Emergency Physicians, Gregory Noll, hazardous materials coordinator of the Prince George's County (Maryland) Fire Department, and E. Kent Gray, Agency for Toxic Substances and Disease Registry, who graciously and constructively reviewed our manuscript; Dr. Richard L. Judd, executive dean at Central Connecticut State University, who first introduced us to Brady Books and then taught us to write in simple declarative sentences; our editor, Claire Merrick of Brady Books, who had confidence in us from the start; Isadora and Nathan Borak, whose concern and support has lasted for longer than I can remember.

Jonathan Borak, M.D.

In the course of seventeen years of emergency response and fire service, many people have influenced my attitudes and teaching techniques. They contributed to my knowledge of fire fighting and hazardous materials and helped to define my role as an instructor. Without their support and contributions I would not have had the opportunity, knowledge, or sense of purpose to have written this book. I would like to acknowledge the following people: Dr. James McGaughey, fire surgeon of the Wallingford, Connecticut, Fire Department, for first introducing me to Dr. Jonathan Borak; John Leahy, Retired Chief of the Pittsburgh, Pennsylvania, Fire Department, and Roger McGary, chief of the Montgomery County, Maryland, Fire Department, to whom I am especially grateful for showing me that teaching is more than knowledge—it is enthusiasm, sincerity, and a genuine love of the fire service; Chief Jack McElfish, Wallingford, Connecticut, Fire Department, for giving me the opportunity and encouragement to grow beyond my local limits; Shift 3, "The Vulture Squad" of the Wallingford Fire Department, for serving as educational "guinea pigs" as I tried out new ideas and teaching styles; Greg Noll, for always being there when I call with questions and unselfishly sharing every bit of information that he has; Frank Docimo, Turn of River Fire Department in Stamford, Connecticut, for all he has done to help me understand both hazardous materials and myself. I may speak or write the words, but the concepts were developed jointly with Frank; Bonnie, Mike, and Matt Callan, three people who make doing this worthwhile. Bonnie deserves most of the credit for anything I have ever done that is good. She has had the patience to bear with me and my difficult schedule. She understands that I love to teach and lets me do it. And she has the courage and fortitude to tell me when I do it too much!

Michael Callan

Along with thanks to our editors, reviewers, and friends who helped to make this book happen, I would like to extend warm acknowledgment to the following people: Charles Raubeson, deputy chief fire marshal of West Haven, Connecticut, for his enormous contributions to the development of EMS in Connecticut and for inspiring me to pursue an EMS career; Chief William S. Johnson, West Haven Central Fire Department, who supported and encouraged me as I developed my interests and commitments to EMS and hazardous materials response; the physicians and paramedic coordinators of South Central Connecticut's EMS community, for sharing the time, knowledge, and concerns necessary to have built a first-class EMS system; Christine Abbott, for giving up her time and career to nurture mine; Colene and Christopher Hawes, for the patience that they showed in dealing with my impatience; my mother, Madaline Borders, to whom I am grateful for many things including her encouragement that I become a teacher.

William Abbott

HAZARDOUS MATERIALS ARE ALL AROUND US

CHAPTER 1

GOAL: On completion of this chapter the student will understand what hazardous materials are, will be able to describe their risks, and will be able to describe possible outcomes at emergencies where hazardous materials are present.

OBJECTIVES:

Specifically, the student will be able to

- Identify the two states in which chemicals exist
- Define the term *hazardous materials*
- Define the term *dangerous goods*

OVERVIEW

It is a fact of life that chemicals, both toxic and benign, are here to stay. An irony of the modern world is that products so essential to our well being also have the potential for such enormous harm.

Chemicals can be thought of as existing in two states or conditions: controlled and uncontrolled (Figure 1–1).

Chemicals in the controlled state act as an essential component in the manufacture of products that contribute to a better way of life. This is the way that we normally expect chemicals to be. In the uncontrolled state, conversely, chemicals can kill and injure people, destroy the environment, and disrupt the normal functions of our communities.

The effects of uncontrolled chemicals, and the emergencies that they cause, have become part of the disaster folklore of our century. We often fail to

1

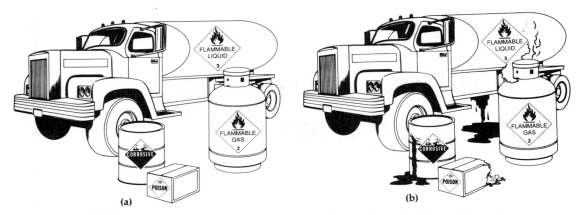

Figure 1–1 Hazardous materials exist in two conditions: (a) controlled and (b) uncontrolled.

remember the names of the chemicals that became uncontrolled and caused havoc and destruction, but we easily recognize the names of the towns and cities that suffered those chemical furies: Texas City, Times Beach, Love Canal, Chernobyl, and Bhopal. The names of those chemical disaster sites are more than familiar to us. They have come to represent the potential destruction that any of us may experience in our own homes and communities as a result of uncontrolled chemical emergencies.

To be prepared to respond to hazardous materials incidents better, emergency responders must first recognize that every community contains potentially hazardous chemicals that exist in the normal, controlled state. Response teams should identify and list the locations where such chemicals are most likely to be found in their own towns and cities. To help begin that process, this chapter will first define hazardous materials, then discuss briefly several concepts of the harm that hazardous materials can cause, and finally it will consider how and where those materials are found in our communities.

DEFINITIONS OF HAZARDOUS MATERIALS

We have just said that chemicals can be controlled or uncontrolled, and that the latter cause emergencies. The potential for danger exists, however, even with controlled chemicals. For example, concentrated acid inside a closed bottle is controlled and poses no actual danger unless it is dropped or spilled. That bottle must be handled with care, however, because of the acid's potential danger. In a similar way, potential danger is posed by tank trucks full of gasoline, 1-ton cylinders filled with chlorine, and properly functioning nuclear reactors even when the hazardous materials in each case are controlled.

We need a definition that goes beyond the concept of control to explain those qualities of certain chemicals that make them potential risks. Technical definitions of the term *hazardous materials* (known as *dangerous goods* in Canada) have been written into governmental policies and legislation, and provide a useful starting point as we gain an understanding of the hazards of chemicals.

One example of such a definition is provided by the U.S. Department of Transportation (DOT). That agency is especially concerned with the dangers posed by chemicals as they move about our communities in trucks, trains, and planes. Their focus is on risks of transportation accidents involving chemical transport vehicles. Accordingly, DOT defines a hazardous material as

> Any substance or material in a quantity or form that poses an unreasonable risk to health, safety, and property when transported in commerce (National Fire Academy, *Recognizing and Identifying Hazardous Materials*, Emmitsburg, Md., p. I-2, 1985).

The usefulness of this definition is, unfortunately, limited. Community responders should be concerned about chemicals that are not necessarily being ''transported in commerce'' and that are used, produced, or stored at local plants or factories. Moreover, the phrase ''unreasonable risk'' is vague. An unreasonable risk to one person (such as mountain climbing or race car driving) need not seem unreasonable to anyone else.

A more useful definition is provided by the U.S. Environmental Protection Agency (EPA), which defines extremely hazardous substances as

> extremely hazardous to the community during an emergency spill or release as a result of its toxicity, and physical and chemical properties. (National Fire Academy, *Recognizing and Identifying Hazardous Materials*, Emmitsburg, Md., p. I-2, 1985).

Although the EPA definition is useful in identifying the scope of hazardous materials that might result in a community disaster, it is difficult for those lacking a solid background in toxicology and chemistry to understand.

An immediately meaningful, albeit less formal, definition of a hazardous material has been coined by Ludwig Benner, hazardous materials specialist with the National Safety Transportation Board. His vivid definition is readily understood without a technical education. According to Benner, a hazardous material is

> Any substance that jumps out of its container at you when something goes wrong and hurts and harms the things it touches (National Fire Academy, *Recognizing and Identifying Hazardous Materials*, Emmitsburg, Md., p. I-2, 1985).

Benner's description of a hazardous material is useful because it identifies a chemical's potential for harm. He provides criteria for identifying hazardous materials that are relevant to the myriad names and titles associated with chemicals today.

HAZARDOUS MATERIALS ARE EVERYWHERE

Look under the kitchen sink for cleaning fluids and drain cleaner, or look around the cellar or garage for old paints and paint thinner. If you know what to look for, you will almost certainly recognize the containers of hazardous materials that share your home with you: flammable liquids, poisons, and corrosives.

Fortunately, most of us keep only small amounts of hazardous chemicals stored in our homes. That does not mean that they cannot cause you harm. To the contrary, even small quantities of insecticides, cleaning solutions, and other such substances can cause injury or death. It is unlikely, however, that these small amounts will pose significant harm to our communities.

By contrast, industrial chemicals pose threats of large-scale damage and destruction. Those chemicals are also all around us. The four hazardous chemicals that most frequently cause harm are gasoline, natural gas, chlorine, and ammonia. They cause harm so often because they are used in large volumes in every community. They are so common, in fact, that we may easily take them for granted and forget the dangers that they pose.

Identifying less common hazardous materials can sometimes be difficult. To facilitate this process, the EPA has been required under federal laws, particularly Superfund (also known as CERCLA, Comprehensive Environmental Response Compensation and Liability Act) and SARA, to publish lists of hazardous and extremely hazardous substances. The formulation of those lists was a necessary first step toward identifying the hazardous risks in our communities. Nearly one thousand separate chemicals have been listed in this way. Many states, counties, and local governments have also enacted similar reporting requirements known as community "right-to-know" laws.

The next step is to locate the sites where those hazardous substances are used, stored, or produced. To assist that process, most industrial users of hazardous chemicals are required under SARA to make lists of the chemicals that they use and provide those lists to community emergency planning councils and emergency responders. In most communities, therefore, emergency planners and responders should now be able to identify the types and locations of hazardous materials that are stored or used in large quantities.

RECOGNITION OF A HAZARDOUS MATERIALS LOCATION

Despite the good intentions of federal legislation, it is likely that hazardous materials incidents will sometimes occur at sites that have not been reported to emergency planners. It is also likely that responders will sometimes be forced to deal with emergencies caused by unknown chemicals. It is essential, therefore, that responders be alert to the possibilities of such emergencies. Early recognition of such possibilities is the single best way to prevent disasters.

Nearly half of all hazardous materials incidents occur at fixed sites where chemicals are normally used, produced, or stored. Under "normal" conditions those chemicals are controlled and pose only potential threat. If emergency responders can identify those sites that use chemicals in a normal, controlled way, then they will also have recognized the sites at which many hazardous chemical accidents could occur.

Some of these sites are easily identified. Factories and chemical plants, for example, are obvious chemical users and producers. Less obvious are storage places, either at plants or warehouses, railroad sidings, and transportation companies. Bulk storage locations may not always be known or well marked. Sometimes only the presence of characteristic 55-gallon drums makes these locations recognizable.

Small industrial sites and commercial companies, such as dry cleaning plants, may be too small to be required to file under the requirements of SARA, yet dangerous quantities of chemicals may be stored there. Likewise, most farms are exempted from the SARA regulations, yet most do contain such hazards as ammonia and flammable liquids. Finally, hazardous materials can often be found, identified or not, in garbage, waste disposal, and other similar locations. Responders must show great care in identifying the possible hazards at these locations before they commit themselves to entry and action (Figure 1–2).

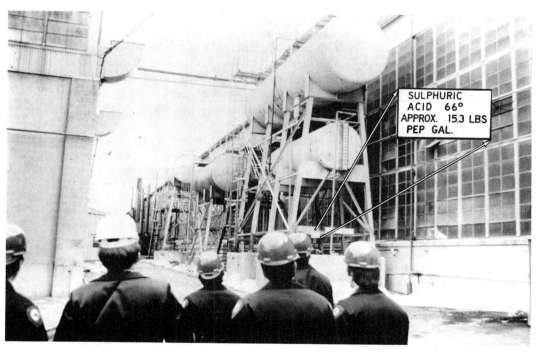

Figure 1–2 Pre-planning is the key to understanding where hazardous materials are in your community. Emergency responders should tour area facilities whenever possible.

More than half of all hazardous materials accidents occur during transport of chemicals. It has been estimated that more than 250,000 shipments of hazardous materials occur daily in the United States. More than 4 billion tons of chemicals are transported annually. Raw products are shipped from producers by rail or truck to manufacturers. Manufactured goods are shipped to retailers for distribution to the end user who discards unused or altered chemicals as wastes that must be carted off to waste dumps and disposal sites. Some chemicals and consumer gases are shipped by pipe line, whereas others are moved about in ships. The fuels that power the means of transportation are all hazardous materials of one form or another.

Transportation is a critical phase in the production and use of hazardous materials; however, it is much more difficult for emergency responders to be prepared for transportation accidents involving hazardous materials. Because of SARA, most emergency response teams can anticipate which chemicals will be found at fixed sites in their communities. It is not possible to have complete knowledge about the chemicals being transported through any community at any given time. Trucks on the highways, for example, may pass through a different community every few minutes. At any given moment, dozens of different tankers and railroad cars may be moving through each city and town.

Large transport tankers and railroad cars containing hazardous chemicals are required to carry placards so that emergency responders will recognize the presence of hazardous materials and their implications. It is critical that emergency responders be able to read and understand available warning signs. More important, however, is the fact that smaller shipments of hazardous materials and illegal shipments of dangerous goods and hazardous wastes may not carry placards, but still can pose enormous risks. Emergency responders must always consider the possibility that any vehicular accident involves a hazardous material.

The responder must always be alert to the possibility of a chemical's presence at the site of any emergency because it is likely that every responder will encounter at some time an unanticipated chemical emergency. Failure to recognize this possibility may cause the responder to become a victim.

THE CONCEPT OF HARM

The potential for harm to victims, spectators, and rescuers is the most important issue that emergency responders must face when confronted with chemicals in the uncontrolled state. Failure to address the potential for harm will often result in additional victims. Too often, these victims are members of the response team who, with the best of intentions, are harmed because of their lack of knowledge, caution, and preplanning.

Safe actions at a hazardous materials incident require information. On arrival at any incident scene, emergency responders must gather the *appropriate* information needed to assess the emergency. Rescuers who are always prepared to confront a hazardous material at any incident are more likely to recognize their presence and take appropriate precautions.

Visual and sensory clues can provide responders with a means for quick assessment of an emergency scene. Consider Figure 1–3. Does it present a hazardous materials incident? Perhaps. Do we need more information to be certain? Absolutely. Should the rescue begin before more information is obtained? No!

The more information about an incident that is available to a response team, the more likely that a safe and healthy outcome will result. For example, consider the additional information needed to understand the problems presented in Figure 1–3. It portrays a scene that could have many alternative underlying plots. To illustrate this point, consider two different stories that might explain Figure 1–3:

1. The scene involves a bakery and the victim is the baker. Witnesses recount that before he fell to the bakery floor he clutched his chest and moaned. The baker was scheduled for coronary bypass surgery in the near future.

2. The scene involves a water treatment plant and the victim was changing chlorine cylinders just before he collapsed to the floor. A strong odor of chlorine is in the room.

Either story could be an accurate description of that scene. In one, a prompt EMS response might save a cardiac victim. In the other, an overly rapid entry might convert rescuers into hazardous materials victims. It is vital that responders who have been trained to provide prompt aid to victims learn to proceed with deliberate caution, anticipate the presence of hazardous materials, and plan their rescue actions according to what they learn about the emergency setting. A deliberate approach can protect the health of rescuers and victims that

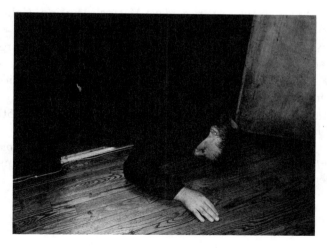

Figure 1–3   Why is this man down?

might otherwise be compromised through well-meant but poorly thought-out actions.

A detailed discussion of the concerns for planning the rescue to assure the safety of emergency responders will be presented in chapter 8.

SUMMARY

The role of emergency responders has never been an easy one. A certain amount of risk and danger always exists. Moreover, it is often necessary to make life-and-death decisions quickly and under difficult circumstances. The presence of hazardous materials makes the responder's job still more difficult.

Obtaining accurate information promptly is a critical first step in a hazardous materials response. Through appropriate preplanning, it is often possible to identify the types and sites of hazardous chemicals that might confront rescuers in any community. Transportation accidents, conversely, are more difficult to plan for and can pose additional hazards to emergency responders.

Emergency response teams must promptly determine whether hazardous materials are present at every incident before they become endangered in their response. They must decide whether their involvement will favorably affect the outcome of the event. A rescue plan should be established for each incident that provides safety to rescuers while also addressing the needs of victims.

REFERENCES

IFSTA, *Hazardous Materials for First Responders* (1st ed.), ed. Gene P. Carlson. Stillwater, Okla.: Fire Protection Publications, Oklahoma State University, 1988.

ISMAN, WARREN E., and GENE P. CARLSON, *Hazardous Materials*, Encino, Calif.: Glencoe Publishing Co., 1980.

NATIONAL FIRE ACADEMY, *Hazardous Materials Incident Analysis*, Emmitsburg, Md.: National Fire Academy, 1985.

NATIONAL FIRE ACADEMY, *Recognizing and Identifying Hazardous Materials*, Emmitsburg, Md.: National Fire Academy, 1985.

NATIONAL FIRE PROTECTION ASSOCIATION, INC. *Fire Protection Handbook* (15th ed.), Quincy, Mass.: National Fire Protection Association, 1981.

NOLL, GREGORY G., MICHAEL S. HILDEBRAND, and JAMES G. YVORRA, *Hazardous Materials Managing the Incident*, Stillwater, Okla.: Fire Protection Publications, Oklahoma State University, 1988.

PRINCIPLES OF HAZARDOUS MATERIALS BEHAVIOR

CHAPTER 2

GOAL: On completion of this chapter the student will have an understanding of the stages of a hazardous materials emergency, and an understanding of the physical states and properties of chemicals that dictate their behavior.

OBJECTIVES:

Specifically, the student will be able to

- Name the four basic initiators of a hazardous materials emergency
- Describe the difference between *potential risk* vs *actual risk*
- Describe the six stages of a hazardous materials emergency
- Describe the three general categories of harm caused by hazardous materials
- Name the three physical states of a released chemical
- Define the following physical properties of hazardous materials:
  - Vapor pressure
  - Boiling point
  - Vapor density
  - Specific gravity
  - Water solubility
  - Expansion ratio

OVERVIEW

The effective control of a chemical emergency is based on a good working understanding of the principles of chemistry. This does not make a chemist out of an

9

emergency responder, but a responder must know how the "enemy" will behave to deal with it effectively. Firefighters cannot successfully fight a house fire until they have studied fire behavior, building construction, and suppression tactics. Emergency medical technicians and paramedics cannot deliver appropriate emergency medical care without a sound knowledge of anatomy and physiology. Similarly, emergency responders cannot begin to deal with hazardous materials emergencies without a basic grasp of chemistry. Knowledge about the behavior of a chemical and the sequential course of its activity when released is crucial to manage an emergency safely and effectively.

INITIATION OF HAZARDOUS MATERIALS INCIDENTS

Something always initiates a hazardous materials emergency. The four basic initiators of such an emergency are the following:

- Human error
- Environmental conditions
- Container flaws or failure
- Equipment failure

Evaluations of accidents of all sorts have led to a popular view that most are due to human error. It has been said, for example, that human error accounts for 88 percent of accidents, 10 percent are due to equipment error, and the final 2 percent are due to "acts of God." An alternative view, developed by Charles Perrow and applicable to many "high-tech" emergencies, argues that many accidents are actually "normal" events that are due to the intensity and design of modern industrial activities. According to that view, it is not human "error" but human limitations that contribute to most accidents. (From Charles Perrow, *Normal Accidents* (New York: Basic Books, Inc., 1984), p. 1.)

STAGES OF A HAZARDOUS MATERIALS EMERGENCY

Hazardous material emergencies don't "just happen." They evolve through a sequence of "stages" that ultimately leads to an unleashing of the potential for harm that characterizes hazardous substances. An emergency can be said to exist once this sequence has been initiated. At that point, the hazardous material's theoretical potential for harm becomes an actual threat. The further along the sequence, the greater is the likelihood that the potential harm will become realized. The goal of an emergency response is to prevent the sequence from fully evolving.

Let us consider a simple example to make this concept clear. Chlorine is a hazardous chemical that can cause severe harm. It is a liquified gas that is usually stored in high-pressure tanks. It is a hazardous material because it poses the potential for harm, but little likelihood exists that it will actually cause harm while it remains contained. In its tank, chlorine poses a *potential* risk, not an actual one, and the simple presence of a tank of chlorine does not pose an emergency.

If a threat exists that the tank will leak and the chlorine will escape, however, then the situation becomes different. Suppose that a fault is in the tank that could cause a leak, or that a fire threatens to explode the tank. Now the chlorine's risk is no longer a potential one. Instead, it poses an *actual* risk, and an emergency exists. The more likely the leak, the greater the emergency. Once a leak occurs, the emergency increases and so does the probability that the chlorine's potential harm will become actual harm resulting in casualties. At any point along the sequence, from threatened release to actual harm, an emergency response may be able to stop the sequence and thereby limit the emergency.

Work by Ludwig Benner and Charles Wright (supervisor of hazardous material training for the Union Pacific System) divided this sequence in the evolution of hazardous materials incidents into six distinct stages or events. They used the techniques of "event analysis," an analytic process that breaks a complex sequence into its smaller component parts (From Ludwig Benner, Jr., *A Textbook for Use In the Study of Hazardous Materials Emergencies* (Oakton, Virginia: Lufred Industries, 1978, p. 12.). The following six stages or events of a hazardous materials incident make up the hazardous materials general behavior model (Figure 2–1):

1. Stress event

2. Breach event

3. Release event

4. Engulfment event

5. Impingement event

6. Harm event

Stress.   Stress refers to the application of forces on the containers in which hazardous materials are stored and leads to strain, deformity, or weakening of the container. Stress is the first step leading to the release of a container's contents. Stress commonly results from mechanical, thermal, or chemical forces or any combination of the three. Once a container has been stressed, an emergency exists.

An example of mechanical stress occurs when a tank truck is in a vehicular accident. The transfer of energy that results from the collision can mechanically stress the tank. Signs of mechanical stress include dents, punctures, and tears of containers.

Extremes of temperature, either hot or cold, can cause thermal stress to a

Stress Event Analysis

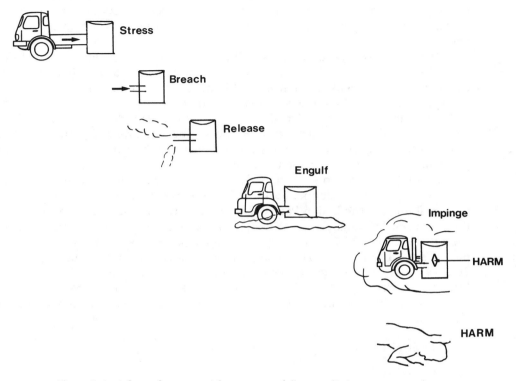

Figure 2–1 A hazardous material emergency follows a distinct sequence of events.

chemical's container. Containers in a fire, for example, can be stressed by the heat as well as by the force of the container's contents, which expand as heat is applied.

Chemical stress results from reactions of chemicals within a container. For example, water entering a chlorine tank reacts with the chlorine and leads to corrosion of the metallic tank.

Breach.   When the stress applied to a container exceeds the container's ability to recover, the container will fail and release its contents. Failure of a container as a result of stress is known as breach. Different types of containers suffer breach in different ways: tanks may be ripped or punctured, cylinders may split, glass bottles can shatter, and bags can tear.

Release.   Once a breach has occurred in a container, its contents are free to be released. The release may be sudden and violent, as when a pressurized tank ruptures or an explosive detonates. Other releases occur slowly, as when a granular insecticide slowly pours out of a torn bag, or a liquid slowly drips from a leak in a small valve or pipe.

Along with hazardous materials, energy may be released from a breached container. This occurs, for example, when an explosion releases heat that can cause harm. Generally the greater the energy released, the more sudden and violent the release event.

At this stage, the goal of emergency response is to limit the volume released and to contain the release before it can cause harm.

Engulfment.   Following release, the hazardous material (or the energy to which that material has been converted) spreads out and disperses. That spread may be rapid or slow. The rate of spread and dispersion is determined by the nature of the hazardous material (is it solid, liquid, or gas?); the type of release that occurred (was it a high-energy explosive release or a low-energy slow release?); and environmental factors (is a strong wind present, or is it raining?).

As it moves, the released materials begin actually to threaten the people, objects, and things in its path. So long as those people and things can escape or be protected, only potential harm exists. Once exposed victims are surrounded—that is, once they have been engulfed—escape is impossible, and actual harm will begin.

At this stage, the goal of emergency response is to evacuate or shelter people and other living things from the path of the released hazard to prevent engulfment.

Impingement.   Impingement occurs when the released hazardous material actually makes contact with people, objects, and things. Impingement can be brief, as when a wave of heat is sent out from an explosion. Impingement can sometimes persist for days or longer, such as when a toxin is released and remains in the atmosphere or water supply. In some cases, impingement can be long term. The radiation accident at Chernobyl, for example, caused radioactive impingement that will likely last for generations.

The process that leads to harm begins at the same time as impingement. Impingement does not always lead to harm, however. The extent of harm that is caused depends in part on the duration of the impingement and the dose of the hazardous material that is received.

At this stage, the goal of emergency response is to minimize the harm that will be caused. It is no longer possible to avoid harm.

Harm.   Harm is the stage of an incident when damage is caused to living things. The types of harm caused depends on the actual hazards released, the way in which the release occurs, and the relationship between the victim and the release. Three general categories of harm caused by hazardous materials are the following:

- Health
- Flammability
- Reactivity

Combinations of these three forms of harm can lead to several different mechanisms of harm including thermal injury, mechanical injury, radioactive injury, toxic injury, corrosive injury, and etiologic or infectious injury. These specific forms of harm will be discussed in more detail in a later chapter (chapter 3).

PHYSICAL PROPERTIES OF HAZARDOUS MATERIALS

The physical state and physical properties of a hazardous material determine the manner in which it spreads and moves following release from its container. Knowledge of the alternative forms and actual properties of a chemical will allow emergency responders to predict its behavior. In turn, this allows responders to control and contain the hazardous material and avoid engulfment.

The *physical state* of a released chemical is either solid, liquid, or gas (Figure 2–2). Gases are able to move most rapidly and pose the greatest threat of sudden engulfment. Liquids are also mobile. They tend to flow downhill and along paths of least resistance. In some situations, droplets of liquids become airborne and form "mists." Mist formation is more common as the environmental temperature and humidity increase, and when the liquid is agitated. Solids are least likely to be moved. Solid dust particles can become airborne, however, and form "fumes" that can act like gases and mists. Solids can also be carried by water and other liquids, such as the run-off from fire hoses, and the shoes and clothing of rescuers and victims who contact the solid.

The physical properties that contribute to the behavior and movement of hazardous materials and that are of greatest importance to emergency responders include the following:

1. Vapor pressure
2. Boiling point
3. Vapor density
4. Specific gravity
5. Water solubility
6. Expansion or liquid-gas ratios

Vapor pressure.   The *vapor pressure* is a measure of the tendency of a liquid to vaporize into a gas. The vapor pressure is dependent on the temperature, increasing as the temperature rises. Standard vapor pressure is usually mea-

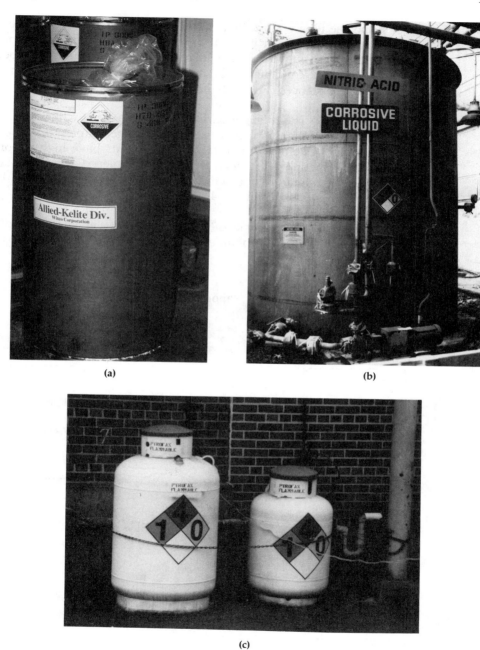

(a)

(b)

(c)

Figure 2–2 Hazardous materials exist in three states: solid, liquid, or gas. (a) Industrial strength cleaner in the form of granules. (b) Nitric acid, a corrosive liquid. (c) Propane gas.

sured at a specific temperature that is equivalent to room temperature (about 68°F). Substances with vapor pressures greater than the standard air pressure at sea level rapidly evaporate. These substances pose particular risks because, once released from a container, they rapidly vaporize and can be carried by winds over large distances (Figure 2–3).

Boiling point.   The *boiling point* is the temperature at which a chemical's vapor pressure equals atmospheric pressure. At that temperature, the liquid rapidly evaporates. Chemicals with low boiling points have high vapor pressures. They are sometimes described as being "volatile." Chemicals that exist as gases at room temperature and standard atmospheric pressure have, by definition, low boiling points (Figure 2–4).

Vapor density.   The *vapor density* is the weight of a given volume of vapor or gas compared to the weight of an equal volume of dry air, both measured at

Vapor Pressure

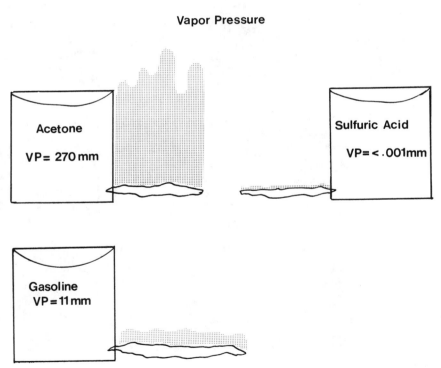

Figure 2–3   The amount of released harmful vapors is based on the chemical's vapor pressure. The greater the vapor pressure, the greater the yield of hazardous vapors. Acetone will give off more vapors than gasoline. Sulfuric acid has a low vapor pressure and gives off little vapor.

Boiling Point

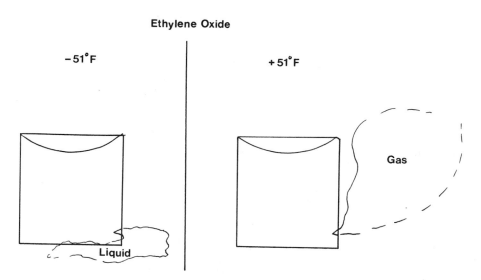

Figure 2-4 Ethylene oxide has a boiling point of 51°F. Below 51°F it is a liquid; above 51°F it boils off into a gas.

the same temperature and pressure. By agreement, the vapor density of air is determined to equal 1. A chemical with a vapor density less than 1 is less dense than air. When released, such a gas will rise and dissipate. Chemicals with vapor densities greater than 1 are denser than air. They tend to settle or sink (Figure 2-5). Most gases are denser than air.

Responders must understand the concept of vapor density because it provides important warning information about where a released chemical is likely to be found. Because most vapors are denser than air, they collect in low areas. Rescuers who enter places that are below grade level (such as cellars and basements, a deep median between the lanes of an interstate highway, or depressions and hollows of an open field) risk being exposed to high concentrations of vapors that have accumulated there.

Specific gravity. The *specific gravity* is the weight of a substance compared to the weight of an equal amount of water. The specific gravity of water is determined to equal 1. A chemical with a specific gravity less than 1 is less dense than water. Such a chemical will tend to float on top of water when poured together. Chemicals with specific gravities greater than 1 are denser than water. They tend to sink to the bottom if mixed with water. Gasoline, for example, has a specific gravity of 0.66 and will float on top of water. Carbon disulfide, by contrast, will sink to the bottom if mixed with water because its specific grav-

Vapor Density

Vapor Density

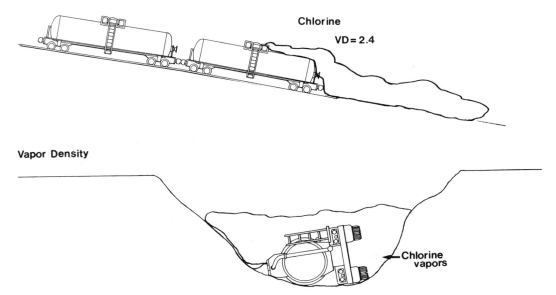

Figure 2–5 The vapor density of a chemical determines the direction in which its vapors will move. Chlorine's vapor density is 2.4; its vapors will flow downhill or accumulate in low-lying areas.

Specific Gravity

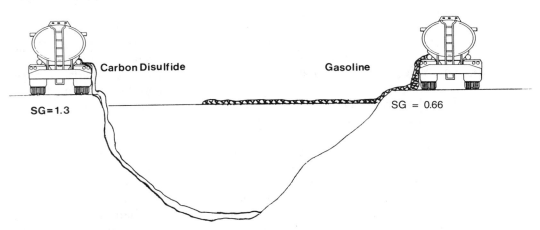

Figure 2–6 Specific gravity is an indication of whether liquids sink or float on water. Carbon disulfide, with a specific gravity of 1.3, will sink. Gasoline, with a specific gravity of 0.66, will float on the surface of water.

ity is 1.3 (Figure 2–6). Chemicals with low specific gravity tend to be quickly spread by moving water because they float on the surface. High specific gravity chemicals tend to sink and are therefore less likely to be widely dispersed by water's effects.

Water solubility.   *Water solubility* is the quantity of a chemical that will mix with or dissolve in water. The water solubility of a chemical helps to determine many of its toxic effects on living tissues. Chemicals that are very water soluble, for example, tend to dissolve in the cell and tissue water of the body, and thereby lead to cellular injury. Water-soluble chemicals can be more easily removed from the skin by washing with water, whereas water-insoluble chemicals may require soap or mild detergent washing to remove them.

The water solubility also determines the effectiveness of water sprays and fogs for containing released chemicals. Those that are water soluble will dissolve in water sprays, thus removing them from the air and limiting their spread. The water run-off from such spraying will then contain large amounts of the dissolved chemical, however, and that water must be contained to prevent the run-off from spreading the hazard (Figure 2–7).

Expansion or liquid-gas ratios.   The *liquid-gas ratio* is the volume of gas produced by the vaporization of a given volume of liquid. The volume of gas produced is always greater than the volume of liquid before vaporization. When this ratio is large, it indicates that a relatively small container of liquid can produce a large volume of gas that may endanger a large area or many people

Water Solubility

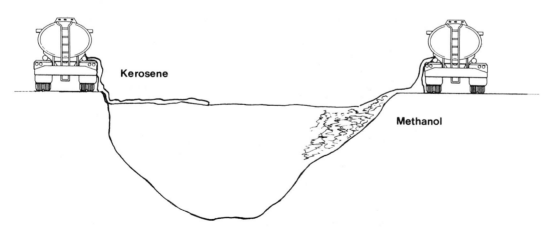

Figure 2–7 Water solubility is a measurement of the ability of a substance to mix with water. Kerosene has a lower solubility measurement and will not mix well. Methanol, like most alcohols, has a high solubility measurement and mixes well with water.

Expansion Ratio

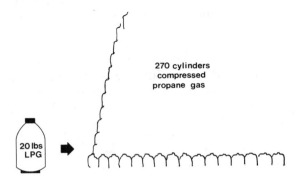

270 cylinders
compressed
propane gas

20 lbs
LPG

Figure 2–8 At an expansion ratio of
270:1, one single 20 lb. cylinder can
produce 270 cylinders filled with
compressed propane gas.

(Figure 2–8). This property is usually presented as a ratio of the form: vapor
volume:liquid volume. The volume of liquid equals 1. For example, the expansion ratio for gasoline is 37:1, which indicates that 1 cubic foot of liquid gasoline
will produce 37 cubic feet of gasoline vapor. The expansion ratio of liquid petroleum is 270:1 and that of liquified oxygen is 700:1.

The expansion ratio of a chemical helps to determine the extent of hazard
that the chemical poses. For example, one reason that chlorine is such a hazard
is that small containers of liquid chlorine can produce large volumes of toxic

Expansion Ratios

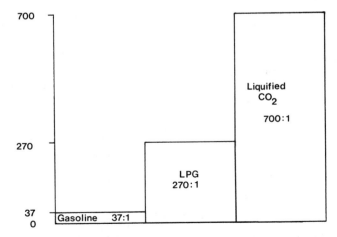

700

Liquified
CO_2

700:1

270

LPG
270:1

37
0

Gasoline   37:1

Figure 2–9 Different chemicals have different expansion ratios. Liquified gases
and cryogenics have the greatest.

chlorine gas. One volume of the liquid forms about 457.6 volumes of gas, and 1 pound of liquid yields about 5 cubic feet of gas. Small storage cylinders contain about 100 to 150 pounds of chlorine and could release about 500 to 750 cubic feet of gas. Typical rail tank cars, by contrast, may contain more than 50 tons of liquid and could generate more than 50 million cubic feet of gaseous chlorine (Figure 2–9).

SUMMARY

Hazardous materials emergencies usually follow a logical sequence of stages. Once that sequence begins, an emergency exists. The goal of emergency response is to prevent the full evolution of the sequence that leads to harm.

Once released, a chemical will move, sometimes with great speed and energy, and sometimes at a slow pace. The state of the substance and its physical properties dictate the behavior of the hazard. Knowledge of the chemical's properties can help responders to anticipate where the hazard can be found, and thereby permit effective avoidance and protective techniques.

REFERENCES

CARLSON, GENE P., ed., *Hazardous Materials for First Responders*. Stillwater, Okla.: Fire Protection Publications, 1988.

ISMAN, WARREN E., and GENE P. CARLSON, *Hazardous Materials*. Encino, Calif.: Glencoe Publishing Co., 1980.

MEYER, EUGENE, *Chemistry of Hazardous Materials*. Englewood Cliffs, N.J.: Prentice-Hall, Inc., 1977.

NATIONAL FIRE ACADEMY, *Hazardous Materials Incident Analysis*. Emmitsburg, Md.: NFA-SM-HMIA/TtT, 1985.

NATIONAL FIRE ACADEMY, *The Pesticide Challenge*. Emmitsburg, Md.: NFA-IG-TPC/TtT, 1985.

NATIONAL FIRE ACADEMY, *Recognizing and Identifying Hazardous Materials*, Emmitsburg, Md.: NFA-SM-RIHM/TtT, 1985.

NATIONAL FIRE PROTECTION ASSOCIATION INC., *Fire Protection Handbook* (15th ed.), Quincy, Mass.: National Fire Protection Association, 1981.

NOLL, GREGORY G., MICHAEL S. HILDEBRAND, and JAMES G. YVORRA, *Hazardous Materials Managing the Incident*. Stillwater, Okla.: Fire Protection Publications, 1988.

PERROW, CHARLES, *Normal Accidents*. New York: Basic Books, Inc., Publishers, 1984.

PRINCIPLES OF HARM CAUSED BY HAZARDOUS MATERIALS

CHAPTER 3

GOAL: On completion of this chapter the student will have an understanding of the basic types of threats that a hazardous material poses to exposure victims.

OBJECTIVES:

Specifically, the student will be able to

- Define flammability
- Define flash point
- Define flammable range
- Define lower explosive limit
- Define upper explosive limit
- Name a chemical with a wide flammable range
- Define autoignition temperature
- Name a chemical with a low autoignition temperature
- Define reactivity
- Name the five groups of hazardous materials that pose particular risk of reactivity harm
- Name two hazardous materials that are water reactive
- Define toxicity
- Define threshold limit value–time-weighted average
- Define permissible exposure limit
- Define threshold limit value–short-term exposure limit
- Define immediately dangerous to life or health
- Define threshold limit value ceiling

OVERVIEW

The potential scope of a hazardous materials emergency is determined in part by the physical properties of the particular materials involved. How large an area will be contaminated and how many people threatened, for example, are directly related to the quantity of chemical involved and the form in which that chemical is found. Those are the considerations that were discussed in the previous chapter.

Of equal or greater importance to rescuers are the actual types of threats that a hazardous material poses to exposure victims. Toxic chemicals and poisons can be harmful in many specific ways, but for general discussion these are usually divided into the following three categories of harm:

- Flammability harm
- Reactivity harm
- Health effect harm

All three forms of harm can be lethal. *Flammability harm* refers to thermal injuries that are caused when hazardous materials ignite and burn. *Reactivity harm* results from the release of energy when hazardous materials undergo chemical reactions. Chemical reactions can lead to explosions that cause severe traumatic injuries. *Health effect harm* includes the many different ways in which chemicals interact with the body's cells to disrupt normal function and cause injury or illness.

These categories of harm tend to overlap. Burn injuries and explosion injuries, for example, can be said to cause negative health effects. Likewise, the release of heat from a burning chemical is one example of a chemical's ''reactivity.'' Nevertheless, the categories provide a useful guideline for classifying the sorts of harm that individual hazardous materials can cause. Figure 3–1 illustrates a chemical, in this case formaldehyde, that poses many hazards.

In this chapter, we will discuss the three categories of harm in more detail. Special attention will be given to ways in which the potential for each type of harm can be described or measured. In chapter 4, the use of these categories will be considered in commonly employed hazardous materials warning systems. The types of health effects that hazardous materials can cause will be considered in chapters 9 and 15 to 18.

FLAMMABILITY

The flammability of a substance is its capacity to ignite and burn rapidly. The more susceptible a substance is to burning, the greater is its threat of flammability harm. Because nearly 65 percent of all hazardous chemicals are flammable, fire is the most frequent danger associated with hazardous materials accidents,

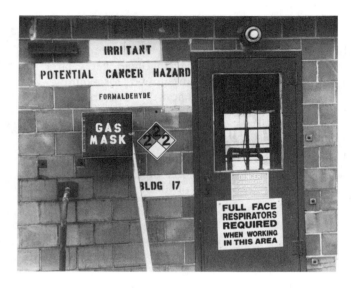

Figure 3–1 A typical example of a chemical that poses many hazards. Formaldehyde threatens flammability, reactivity, and health harm.

and flammability is the most commonly occurring of the three categories of harm.

Emergency responders must be able to evaluate the flammability threat of a hazardous materials accident quickly. To accomplish that, the following concepts and definitions must first be understood:

- Flash point
- Flammable and explosive range
- Autoignition temperature

Flash Point

Nearly all chemicals must be in the gaseous state to burn. Flammable chemicals that exist as gases under standard conditions (such as hydrogen, methane, and propane) can be ignited just as they are. Liquids and solids, conversely, must be vaporized before ignition can occur. For example, imagine an ordinary table candle made of solid wax. To light that candle, it is necessary to vaporize some of the wax. That is usually done by applying heat from a lighted match. At first, heat causes the wax to melt. Then some of the molten wax vaporizes. Finally, the vapors ignite and create the candle's flame. A similar process of vapor formation occurs whenever flammable liquids (such as gasoline and carbon disulfide) or flammable solids (such as wax and cadmium) are ignited.

Flash point is the term used to describe the minimum temperature at which a substance gives off enough vapor to ignite when exposed to a spark or flame. At the flash point, the quantity of vapors will support a ''flash'' of burning, but it will not continue to burn. Continuous burning requires larger quantities of vapors that can form at only temperatures that are greater than the flash point.

The fire hazard of a substance is related to its flash point. The lower the flash point, the easier it is to form flammable vapors. Chemicals with flash points below standard room temperature are usually dangerous fire hazards. Unlike the candle described earlier, low flash point substances do not require heat to produce flammable vapors. Such vapors form at room temperature whenever their containers are left open. Two examples of low flash point chemicals that pose important fire hazards are gasoline (flash point of −45°F) and carbon disulfide (flash point of −22°F).

Emergency responders at a chemical accident must know that if a spilled chemical has a flash point that is lower than the temperature of the contaminated place, then the chemical poses a significant risk of fire and flammability harm.

Flammable (Explosive) Range

The flash point is not the only determinant of fire hazard. Another important factor involves the concentration of flammable vapor in the air of the contaminated place. As the vapor forms, it mixes with oxygen in the air. If enough flammable vapor is not available, or if too much vapor exists and not enough oxygen is present, then ignition will be impossible. The *flammable (explosive) range* describes the range of vapor concentration in air that will burn or explode if ignited. That range is described in terms of the volume percentage of the vapor in air.

For each chemical, a specific flammable (explosive) range exists in which the vapors are readily ignited. The range is defined by ''upper'' and ''lower'' limits. Below the lower limit, often called the *lower explosive limit* (LEL), enough vapor is not available to burn. The mixture of air and vapor is too ''lean.'' Above the upper limit, often called the *upper explosive limit* (UEL), the mixture of air and vapor is too ''rich.'' Too much vapor exists, and not enough oxygen is present (Figure 3–2).

The concept of flammable (explosive) range can be explained by analogy to the carburetor of an automobile. If the carburetor is set so that too little gasoline enters the engine, then the gasoline cannot ignite, and the car will not run. Such a carburetor setting is too lean. Conversely, if too much gasoline enters the engine, then the engine will not run because too little oxygen exists to burn the fuel. In this example, the carburetor is set too rich. The flammable (explosive) range of a chemical is equivalent to the range of carburetor settings that will allow the engine to run.

It is important to recognize that although vapor concentrations above the UEL will not ignite, they are unsafe. At some future time, that vapor concentration must fall, probably as a result of ventilation of the contaminated place and dissipation of the vapors. When that happens, the ''too rich'' concentration will

LEL/UEL

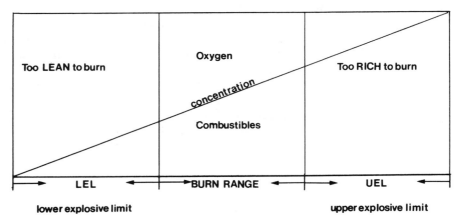

Figure 3-2 A specific concentration exists at which vapors will burn. This concentration has a minimum value (lower explosive limit [LEL]) and a maximum value (upper explosive limit [UEL]).

fall into the flammable range, and it will then pose an important fire hazard. Emergency responders must remember that the ''safety'' of vapor concentrations greater than the flammability range may be temporary.

Some chemicals have narrow flammable ranges, whereas others have wide ranges. In general, the wider the flammability range, the more dangerous is the fire hazard of the chemical. The ranges for several commonly used chemicals are presented in Table 3-1. It can be seen that ethylene oxide is an especially great fire hazard because it can never be too rich to ignite. This chemical's ignition could theoretically occur within a closed container. Fortunately, few chemicals pose such flammability risks.

Autoignition Temperature

The formation of flammable vapors at temperatures above the flash point and their accumulation at concentrations within the flammable (explosive) range do not assure that ignition and fire will occur. In most cases, the addition of heat must also exist for ignition to occur. The source of heat can be a spark, an open flame, or even a hot piece of metal. When a heat source comes into contact with an appropriate concentration of flammable vapors, ignition occurs. Ignition can also result from autoignition or spontaneous combustion.

If a flammable substance is heated enough, it will ignite even when no open flame or spark provokes burning. For each flammable chemical a threshold temperature exists at which it will spontaneously ignite. That temperature is called the *autoignition (or ignition) temperature*. Once the autoignition temperature

TABLE 3–1 FLAMMABLE (EXPLOSIVE) RANGES
OF COMMONLY USED CHEMICALS

Chemical	Lower explosive limit (%)	Upper explosive limit (%)
Gasoline	1.7	7.6
Acetone	2.6	12.6
Carbon disulfide	1.3	50.0
Ethylene oxide	3.0	100.0

has been reached, a self-sustaining combustion will occur that is independent of other heat sources.

Hazardous substances with low autoignition temperatures pose greater flammability risks and dangers than those with higher thresholds. Phosphorus, for example, spontaneously ignites at temperatures above 86°F to 90°F. Because this autoignition temperature is lower than normal body temperature, anyone touching phosphorus can ignite it and be burned. By contrast, the autoignition temperature of carbon disulfide is 212°F, and gasoline's is 982°F.

REACTIVITY

Reactivity refers to the ability of a substance to undergo transformation or change as a result of interactions with air, water, and other chemicals or extinguishing agents, causing a release of energy. Harm results from the sudden impact of that energy. The most dramatic example of reactivity is an explosion that comes about when two incompatible chemicals (for example, formaldehyde and strong acids) are mixed together. Many chemicals can yield large amounts of energy following reactions with other substances. Emergency responders should recognize the following five groups of hazardous chemicals that pose particular risk of reactivity harm:

- Explosives
- Air-reactive materials
- Water-reactive materials
- Unstable monomers
- Hypergolic materials

Explosives are compounds that are unstable and break down with the sudden release of large amounts of energy. They are categorized according to the quantity of energy that can be released. As described in chapter 4, explicit labeling is required when any quantity of the most potent explosives, (categorized as class A and class B explosives) are transported. Less potent explosives (class

C and blasting agents) are capable of great harm but only when found in large quantities. Explosions can also occur when strongly incompatible chemicals are mixed together and when unstable monomers spontaneously polymerize.

Air-reactive materials are substances with low autoignition temperatures. These substances are generally unable to ignite while contained, because under such conditions they produce vapor concentrations in excess of their UEL. Once released, however, they spontaneously and suddenly ignite. These compounds are sometimes called *pyrophoric materials*. Examples of such hazardous substances include phosphorus and aluminum alkyls.

Water-reactive materials are substances that violently react with water to release energy. Such chemicals can pose special problems in situations in which use of water by emergency responders is otherwise routine. For example, copious washing with water is the treatment of choice for most chemical skin exposures. Washing with water should not be used, however, for the management of skin exposure to alkali metals (such as sodium and magnesium), because those metals react with water. When these chemicals come into contact with water, heat and corrosive materials are produced. As a result, skin washing leads to more severe skin injuries.

It is important that water-reactive chemicals be quickly recognized so that water is not used on them. This is particularly relevant for firefighters, who could cause violent explosions if they applied water to fires involving water reactive chemicals. Figure 3-3 illustrates the characteristic symbol used to label water reactive substances.

Unstable monomers are highly reactive chemicals that are normally used in the production of synthetic fibers and plastics. Their industrial value comes from their ability to form long chains called *polymers*, which consist of many monomer molecules joined together. The industrial processes by which monomers join to form polymers yields large amounts of energy and heat, and must be carefully controlled. If monomers are exposed to excess heat, sunlight, contamination, or certain chemical stimuli, they can polymerize spontaneously and violently. This

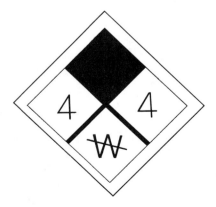

Figure 3-3 This symbol is the one most frequently used for indicating *dangerous when wet* or *use water cautiously*.

may occur while the monomers are still in their containers and can lead to violent explosions.

Hypergolic materials ignite spontaneously on contact with one another without requiring a source of ignition. This quality is highly valued in rocket fuels. An example of hypergolic materials are hydrazine and nitrogen dioxide, a combination that is used as a rocket fuel for maneuvering the National Aeuronautics and Space Administration's space shuttle while outside of the earth's atmosphere.

HEALTH EFFECTS

Persons who make contact with hazardous materials may experience a spectrum of negative health effects because the chemicals interfere with normal functioning of the body's cells. This ability of a chemical to cause harm is known as its *toxicity.* Various specific mechanisms by which chemicals cause toxic harm are discussed later in chapters 9 and 15 to 18.

Safety standards have been established as guidelines to prevent workers and others from exposure to large amounts of hazardous chemicals that can cause toxic harm. Some of these standards have been set by the government, some by industry, and others by independent groups of medical and industrial hygiene professionals. In some cases, standards have been set to prevent exposures that can lead to serious injury or illness. In other cases, the limits are intended to prevent lesser health effects such as irritation of eyes or skin. Figure 3–4 is OSHA's target organ categorization of health effects that may occur, including examples of signs and symptoms and chemicals that have caused such effects.

It is important that emergency responders recognize and understand the standards and commonly used units of measure that indicate the relative toxicity of hazardous materials. These standards and exposure limits are usually stated in terms of the maximum concentration of a chemical to which a person can be safely exposed during a specified length of time. The concentrations of chemicals are usually measured in parts per million (ppm) or milligrams per cubic meter of air (mg/cu meter) (Figure 3–5).

The following are five of the most commonly used exposure limits and measures of the relative toxicity of hazardous materials. These exposure limits and measures refer to a chemical's concentration in air and the duration of exposure; they establish concentration limits that are intended to prevent the development of health effect harm or toxicity.

Threshold Limit Value–Time-Weighted Average (TLV/TWA)

The *TLV/TWA* is the maximum average concentration (averaged over 8 continuous hours) to which an otherwise healthy adult can be repeatedly and safely

OSHA'S TARGET ORGAN CATEGORIZATION OF HEALTH EFFECTS
OF HAZARDOUS MATERIALS

a. Hepatotoxins:
Signs and Symptoms:
Chemicals:

Chemicals which produce liver damage.
Jaundice; liver enlargement.
Carbon tetrachloride; nitrosamines.

b. Nephrotoxins:
Signs and Symptoms:
Chemicals:

Chemicals which produce kidney damage.
Edema; proteinuria.
Halogenated hydrocarbons; uranium.

c. Neurotoxins:

Signs and Symptoms:

Chemicals:

Chemicals which produce their primary toxic
effects on the nervous system.
Narcosis; behavioral changes; decrease in motor
functions.
Mercury; carbon disulfide.

d. Agents which act on the blood or hematopoietic
system:
Signs and Symptoms:
Chemicals:

Decrease hemoglobin function; deprive the body
tissues of oxygen.
Cyanosis; loss of consciousness.
Carbon monoxide; cyanides.

e. Agents which damage the lung:

Signs and Symptoms:
Chemicals:

Chemicals which irritate or damage the
pulmonary tissue.
Cough, tightness in chest; shortness of breath.
Silica; asbestos.

f. Reproductive toxins:

Signs and Symptoms:
Chemicals:

Chemicals which affect the reproductive
capabilities including chromosomal damage
(mutations) and effects on fetuses
(teratogenesis).
Birth defects; sterility.
Lead; DBCP.

g. Cutaneous hazards:

Signs and Symptoms:
Chemicals:

Chemicals which affect the dermal layer of the
body.
Defatting of the skin; rashes, irritation.
Ketones, chlorinated compounds.

h. Eye hazards:
Signs and Symptoms:
Chemicals:

Chemicals which affect the eye or visual capacity.
Conjunctivitis; corneal damage.
Organic solvents; acids.

Figure 3–4 The Occupational Safety and Health Administration's target organ categorization of the health effects of hazardous materials.

exposed for periods of 8 hours per day, 40 hours per week. The duration of exposure is intended to be equivalent to a normal work week. This measurement is established by the American Council of Governmental and Industrial Hygienists (ACGIH), and is important for the regulation of long-standing exposure to chemicals in the workplace. It is primarily intended as an exposure guide rather than as an absolute exposure limit.

CARBON MONOXIDE

TIME	X	CONCENTRATION	=	DOSE EFFECT
2-3 hrs	x	200 ppm	=	Mild Effects (mild headache, nausea)
5-min	x	3,200 ppm	=	Moderate Effects (severe headache, possible angina)
10-min	x	6,400 ppm	=	Severe Effects (death)
1-3 min	x	12,800 ppm	=	Severe Effects (death)

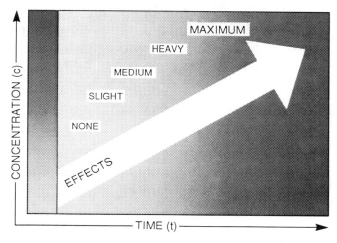

Figure 3–5 Dose is related to either the length of the exposure (time) or the amount of the chemical (concentration). As each increases, the potential for harmful effects increases.

Permissible Exposure Limit (PEL)

The *PEL* is the maximum average concentration (averaged over 8 continuous hours) to which 95 percent of otherwise healthy adults can be repeatedly and safely exposed for periods of 8 hours per day, 40 hours per week. The PEL is established by OSHA and is similar in concept to the TLV/TWA developed by ACGIH. Like the TLV/TWA, PEL is important for the regulation of long-standing workplace exposure to chemicals. It is primarily intended as an exposure guide rather than as an absolute exposure limit.

Threshold Limit Value–Short-Term Exposure Limit (TLV/STEL)

The *TLV/STEL* is the maximum average concentration (averaged over a continuous 15-minute period) to which an otherwise healthy adult can be safely exposed for up to 15 minutes continuously. Workers should not be exposed to the TLV/STEL more than four times per day with at least 60 minutes between each exposure. This measurement is established by the ACGIH and is important for the regulation of acute workplace exposure to chemicals.

Immediately Dangerous to Life or Health (IDLH)

The *IDLH* is that concentration that poses an immediate danger to the life or health of a person who is exposed, but from which the person could escape without any escape-impairing symptoms or irreversible health effects. Concentrations above this limit will cause life or health risks and also impair the ability to escape. This limit is established jointly by OSHA and the National Institute of Occupational Safety and Health (NIOSH). It is important for the regulation of acute workplace exposures to chemicals and serves as a critical criteria for emergency responders planning rescues at hazardous materials incidents.

Threshold Limit Value-Ceiling (TLV-C)

The *TLV-C* is the maximum concentration to which a healthy adult can be exposed without risk of injury.

Exposure to higher concentrations must not occur. This measurement is established by the ACGIH and is similar in concept and use to the IDLH limit developed by NIOSH and OSHA.

CONCEPTS OF SAFETY

By the nature of their work, emergency responders cannot entirely avoid the risks associated with hazardous materials accidents. The responder's goal, therefore, must be to minimize those risks. Achieving that goal requires an understanding of the principles of harm caused by hazardous materials and the various ways that these threats can be mitigated. Ultimately, the safety of the rescue team depends on the quality and scope of information that is available.

To assess the risks of harm that they face, emergency response personnel must first recognize the presence of hazardous materials at an incident. Personnel must then determine the identity of those materials. Therefore, recognition and identification are a necessary first step in developing a safety-oriented response plan. Recognition and identification of hazardous materials are the subjects of chapter 4.

Once the incident hazards have been identified, it is necessary to determine the nature of the threats that each poses. By means of standard reference materials and other data sources (see chapter 5), responders can quickly find the information that describes or measures the flammability, reactivity, and health effect threats of each of those hazards. That information allows response personnel to determine whether they face any threats and which types of threats are most likely.

For responders to know that they are confronted by actual threats of harm, they must measure the concentrations of chemicals in the area of contamination. As explained in chapter 6, measurements of those concentrations can be made with various types of detection instruments. By means of such measurements, the threat of harm at a hazardous materials incident can be objectively evaluated. For example, the probability of fire or explosion can be assessed by knowing the air concentration of a combustible gas, its flammable range, flash point, and the temperature of the contaminated place. Likewise, the likelihood of toxicity can be judged in light of whether any chemical is present at a concentration in excess of its IDLH, TLV/STEL or TLV-C levels.

Once all of this information has been gathered, a response and rescue plan can be developed that does not expose response personnel to unnecessary and unreasonable risks. The choice of personal protective equipment, for example, depends on this full sequence of data gathering (see chapter 7). The same information also provides the basis for determining the most appropriate response to victims (see chapter 8).

If adequate information cannot be obtained, and responders are unable to determine fully the nature of the threats that they will face, then they must act as though they were confronted by a worst-case situation. For example, if the identity or concentration of a toxic chemical cannot be determined, then responders should protect themselves and carry out rescues as though air concentrations exceeded the IDLH and TLV-C levels. When in doubt, response personnel should choose the most conservative approach and practice the highest level of incident safety.

SUMMARY

Exposure to hazardous materials can cause three general types of harm: flammability harm caused by the release of heat, usually owing to burning of the material; reactivity harm caused by the release of energy when chemicals react, often leading to explosions; and health effect harm resulting from the toxic actions of chemicals.

Emergency responders must become familiar with the ways in which a chemical's potential for harm are measured, and the terminology and meaning of various exposure limits. Without an understanding of these concepts, responders may be unable to evaluate adequately the dangers of a hazardous materials incident and, therefore, may become dangerously exposed.

REFERENCES

BRESNITZ, E., K. REST, and N. MILLER: "Clinical Industrial Toxicology: An Approach to Information Retrieval," *Ann. Intern. Med.*, 103 (1985), 967–972.

CARLSON, GENE P., ed., *HazMat Response Team Leak and Spill Guide.* Stillwater, Okla.: Fire Protection Publications, 1984.

LAUWERYS, R. R.: "Occupational Toxicology," in *Casarett and Doull's Toxicology: The Basic Science of Poisons*, pp. 902–15, eds. C. D. KLAASSEN, M. O. AMDUR and J. DOULL. New York: Macmillan Publishing Co., Inc., 1986.

NOLL, G. G., M. S. HILDEBRAND, and J. G. YVORRA: *Hazardous Materials: Managing the Incident.* Annapolis, Md.: Peake Productions, 1988.

PARMEGGIANI, L., ed., *Encyclopedia of Occupational Health and Safety.* Geneva: International Labour Office, 1983.

PROCTOR, N. H., and J. P. HUGHES: *Chemical Hazards of the Workplace*, pp. 3–9. Philadelphia: J.B. Lippincott Company, 1978.

ZAPP, J. A.: "Industrial Toxicology: Retrospect and Prospect," in *Patty's Industrial Hygiene and Toxicology (vol. 2A)*, pp. 1467–91, eds. G. D. CLAYTON, and F. E. CLAYTON. New York: John Wiley & Sons, Inc., 1981.

RECOGNITION AND IDENTIFICATION OF HAZARDOUS MATERIALS

CHAPTER 4

GOAL: On completion of this chapter the student will have an understanding of the clues that should make responders aware of the presence of hazardous materials, and be able to describe warning and labeling systems available to responders.

OBJECTIVES:

Specifically, the student will be able to

- Name the three-step sequence of informational concerns that are critical to the development of appropriate response plans
- Identify the general clues that can lead responders to suspect that an emergency may involve a hazardous material
- Name at least four types of facilities where hazardous materials are commonly used
- Name at least three types of container configurations that are clues to the presence of hazardous materials
- Name the nine hazard classes for placards and labels
- Name the major hazards of each class
- Name the seven symbols that identify types of hazards
- Name the agency responsible for regulating the use of placards and labels
- Name the five classes of hazards for which placards are required regardless of quantity
- Name the title of shipping paper used for rail transportation of hazardous materials
- Name the three types of risks and their accompanying colors addressed by the National Fire Protection Association 704 Marking System

OVERVIEW

Hazardous materials are often present at accident sites and emergency settings. That should not be surprising because hazardous materials are found at places throughout our communities, especially commercial work sites and heavily used transportation routes. It is important for emergency responders to consider the presence of such materials and determine whether they contribute to the emergency or accident. A rescue plan cannot be developed, and the rescue should not be carried out until that information has been determined (see chapter 8).

This chapter is concerned with the recognition and identification of hazardous materials at accident sites. First we will review the clues that should make responders aware of their presence. Then we will discuss some warning and labeling systems that are used so that chemicals in their containers can be correctly identified. Emergency responders should become familiar with these systems to protect themselves and the victims of these incidents better.

RECOGNITION, IDENTIFICATION, AND DETERMINATION OF ROLE

A three-step sequence of informational concerns must be addressed by those involved in emergency response to hazardous materials. These concerns are critical to the development of appropriate response plans and for the protection of involved rescuers. In some cases, the necessary information will be available to responders at the time of dispatch to the emergency. In other cases, no information will be available until rescuers reach the accident scene. In any event, information should be collected as soon as possible.

The first and most basic issue is *recognition* of the presence of a hazardous material. Prompt recognition and awareness of hazardous materials is important for the safety of responders. Without that information, rescuers may fail to take appropriate precautions and enter a contaminated environment without protection.

Identification follows recognition. Once the presence of hazardous materials has been determined, its specific identity and characteristics can be established. Identity of the hazards can lead to more specific management of exposure victims. It also permits more effective containment of the hazardous material and mitigation (that is, selection of spill absorbents) of the incident.

In *determination of the role,* it is necessary to determine whether a hazardous material is playing an active role and contributing to an incident. At many accident scenes, containers of hazardous materials will be innocent bystanders, who are present but not actively part of the incident. For example, most accidents at chemical plants are not caused by chemical releases and do not lead to toxic exposures. Until it has been determined that hazardous materials are not responsible for the injuries or damage at such an accident, however, responders should take actions to protect themselves from exposure.

CLUES TO RECOGNITION

Recognition of the presence of hazardous materials is based on suspicion. Several "clues" can lead emergency responders to suspect the possibility that an incident involves hazardous materials.

Location of the Emergency

Nearly half of all hazardous materials incidents occur at sites where chemicals are manufactured, stored, or used. In most communities, those sites are well known. In many cases, the plants and facilities are required to file lists of their hazardous chemicals with local emergency planning committees and emergency response services. Accordingly, it is often possible to know in advance the actual chemical used at the site of an emergency.

Even without prior knowledge, it is usually easy to recognize those facilities where chemicals are commonly used and found. Accidents at those sites should always raise the suspicion that a hazardous materials incident may be happening. Obvious examples of such facilities include the following:

- Manufacturing plants
- Pharmaceutical companies
- Plastics producers
- Storage facilities and tank farms
- Fuel terminals
- Research facilities
- Gas stations and dry cleaning stores

Refer to Figure 4–1 for some common locations of hazardous materials.

Many hazardous materials incidents result from transportation accidents. Shipments of chemicals are most likely to be found on major highways and large railroad lines, in commercial harbors, and at airports. When responders are dispatched to such locations, they should immediately begin a search for other clues to hazardous materials.

Container Configuration

Chemicals are usually transported and stored in standardized containers. When arriving at an emergency scene, the responder should be aware of the presence of these telltale containers that warn of the presence of chemicals (Figure 4–2). For example, a responder may notice 55-gallon drums and chemical cylinders. A responder may also be dispatched to the scene of an accident involving box cars, tank cars, or over-the-road tankers. Responders should become familiar with the shapes of these containers. See Figure 4–2 for several examples of containers.

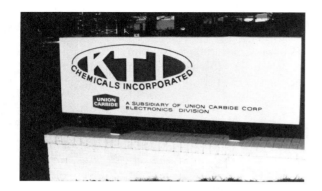

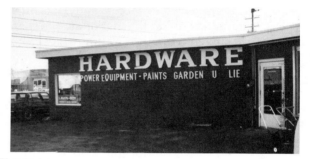

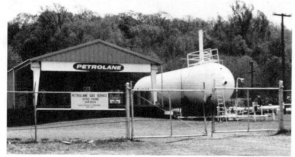

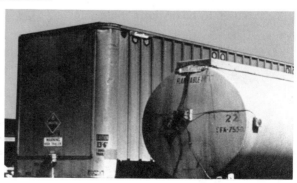

Figure 4–1 Hazardous materials can be found in every community.

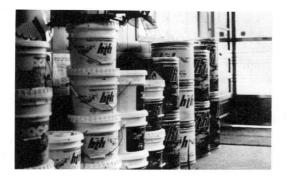
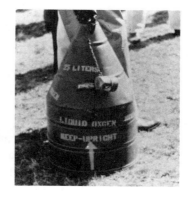
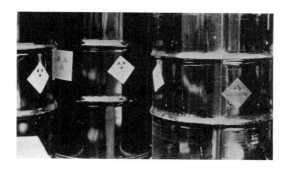
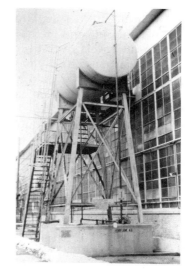
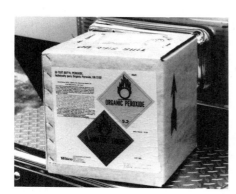
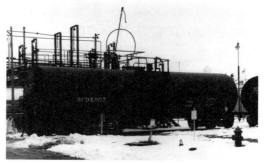

Figure 4–2 Hazardous materials are stored in many types of containers.

Often, containers carry labels or placards that provide specific information about the chemicals they contain. The presence of warning labels should indicate to responders that the contents of the labeled container may pose a hazardous risk. The specific symbols and codes used for placards and labels are discussed later in this chapter.

Sensory Clues

The release of a chemical from its container may be associated with sensory indications that the chemical has escaped into the environment. This may take the form of a visible vapor cloud; a strong or characteristic odor; or irritation caused to the eyes, nose, or throat. Some chemicals provoke sensory reactions at levels that are not harmful. Such chemicals are regarded as having "good warning properties" (for example, chlorine and ammonia). Others (such as vinyl chloride and methanol) have warning properties that are not perceived until unsafe levels have been achieved. A third group (including carbon monoxide and carbon dioxide) have no warning properties at all.

Rescuers should not depend on sensory warning properties to determine the presence of toxic hazards. In some cases, those properties may not be perceived. For example, cyanide has a characteristic odor of bitter almonds, but the ability to smell that odor is a genetic trait, and 20 to 40 percent of people cannot perceive it. In other cases, odor perception may be quickly lost. Hydrogen sulfide, for example, is a lethal gas that smells like rotten eggs. Although its odor is distinctive and perceived at low levels, the ability to perceive it is lost after exposure progresses. Rescuers cannot tell whether the loss of odor indicates a decreased amount of hydrogen sulfide or the start of its toxicity.

In some cases, the presence of sensory clues can help to determine the amount of danger that is present. It is almost always true, for example, that visible vapor clouds occur at chemical concentrations that are well above those that are harmful to living things. Rescuers must not enter or be engulfed by vapor clouds unless they are using appropriate protective equipment (see chapter 7).

CHEMICAL IDENTIFICATION

Recognition warns us that a hazardous material is present at an accident scene. That information is enough to warn responders to take general precautions to prevent exposure. To understand the nature of an emergency and to plan a rescue, it is necessary to obtain more information. Every effort should be made to identify the hazard specifically.

The simplest approach to identification is based on systems of warnings and labels that are placed on bulk and nonbulk containers of hazardous materials. By learning to read and interpret these labels, rescuers can quickly identify the hazards in those containers. In addition to placards and labels, several types of shipping papers and other written documents may be available to emergency responders and serve to identify specific chemicals. These systems and types of documents are discussed subsequently.

A more complex approach to identification is needed when chemicals have been released from unmarked containers or when identification papers are unavailable or have been destroyed. One method involves the use of detection instruments that measure the presence and quantity of chemicals in the air. The use of detection instruments will be discussed in a later chapter (see chapter 6).

Placards and Labels

Placards and labels are placed on chemical containers to convey information about the chemicals within. *Placards* are square diamonds 10¾ inches on each side. *Labels* are smaller square diamonds about 4 inches or smaller on each side. Placards and labels transmit information by means of a series of numbers, symbols, and colors that serve to identify the contained chemical. In some cases, placards and labels identify specific chemicals, whereas in others they serve only to identify the class to which the chemical belongs.

The use of placards and labels and the information that they contain are regulated in the United States by the DOT. Similar systems have been developed in Canada, Europe, and by the United Nations (UN). For the purposes of placarding and labeling, the UN and DOT divide hazardous materials into nine specific classes. Those nine hazard classes are listed in Table 4–1.

Most of these nine hazard classes are further subdivided according to the characteristics within each class. A full listing of the hazard classes and subclasses along with definitions and examples for each is presented in Appendix 1.

The presence of a placard or label tells an emergency responder that the contents of a container are hazardous. Information about the specific characteris-

TABLE 4–1 GENERAL CATEGORIES OF THE UNITED NATIONS AND U.S. DEPARTMENT OF TRANSPORTATION HAZARDS

Class	Category
1	Explosives and blasting agents
2	Pressurized gases
3	Flammable and combustible liquids
4	Flammable solids
5	Oxidizers and organic peroxides
6	Poisonous and infectious substances
7	Radioactive materials
8	Corrosives
9	Other regulated materials

TABLE 4-2 COLOR CODING FOR PLACARDS AND LABELS

Color	Hazard class	Hazard type
Orange	1	Explosives
Red	2–4	Flammables
Green	2	Nonflammable gas
White and red stripes	4	Flammable solid
Yellow	5	Oxidizers/peroxides
White	6	Poisons
Yellow over white	7	Radioactive
White over black	8	Corrosives
White (blank)	9	Other regulated material

tics of that material is provided through a system of colors, symbols, and numbers. There are eight colors or sets of colors that are used for placarding. These are listed in Table 4-2. Examples of colored placards are presented in Fig. 4-3.

Symbols are commonly found on placards. In most cases, these symbols are universally recognized indicators of hazards and dangers. Table 4-3 describes the symbols and their meaning. The symbols themselves are presented in Figure 4-3.

In addition to colors and symbols, placards and labels often contain numbers that identify the labeled chemical. The UN or DOT hazard class number may be printed in the lower corner of the diamond. A system of four-digit numbers has been assigned to specific hazardous chemicals. That system, known as UN or North American identification numbers, must be included on the placards and labels of all chemicals for which such numbers have been assigned. Some UN numbers apply to specific chemicals (for example, number 1086 identifies vinyl chloride), whereas others apply to groups of chemicals with similar hazards (number 1993 indicates a combustible liquid and is used for kerosene, fuel oil, and similar products). This is illustrated in Figure 4-4.

Required use.   In the United States, the use of placards and labels is regulated by the DOT. Requirements for placards are based on the dangers posed

TABLE 4-3 SYMBOL CODING FOR PLACARDS AND LABELS

Symbol	Hazard class	Hazard type
Bursting ball	1	Explosives
Flame	2–4	Flammables
Cylinder	2	Nonflammable gas
"O" with flames	5	Oxidizers
Skull and crossbones	6	Poisons
Propeller	7	Radioactive substances
Tipped test tube	8	Corrosives

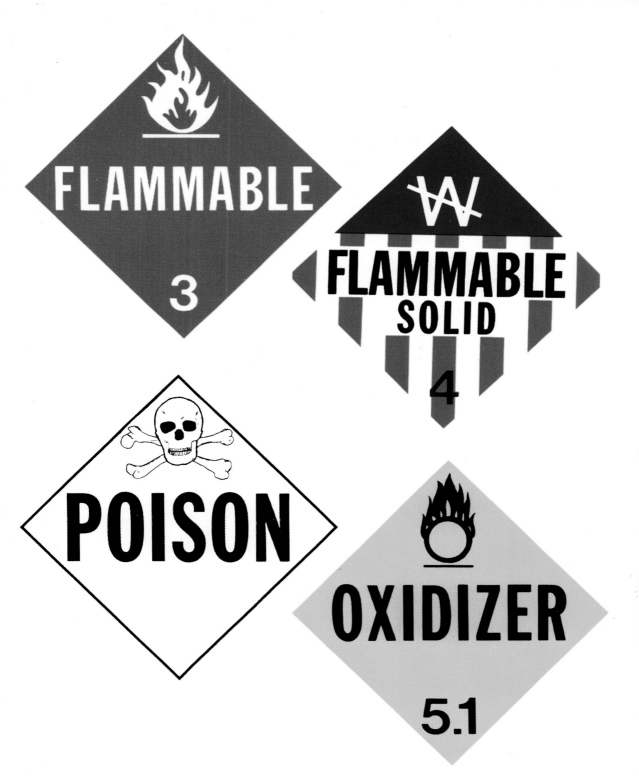

Figure 4–3 The U.S. Department of Transportation symbol coding for placards and labels.

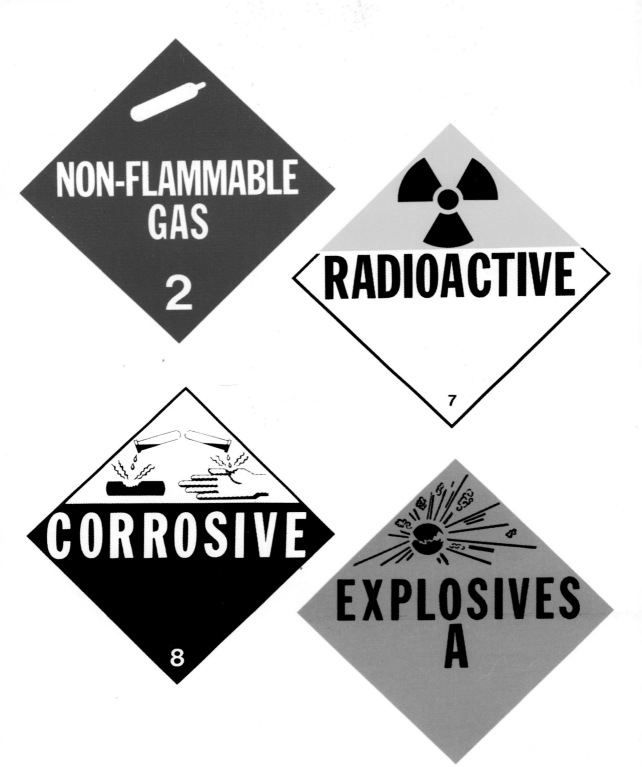

Figure 4–3 *(continued)*

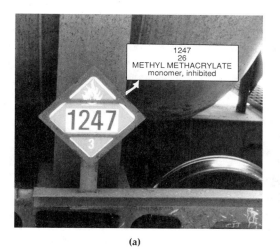

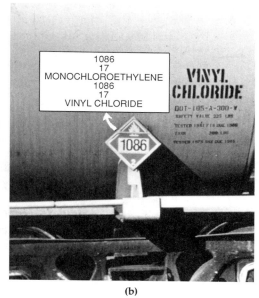

(a)

(b)

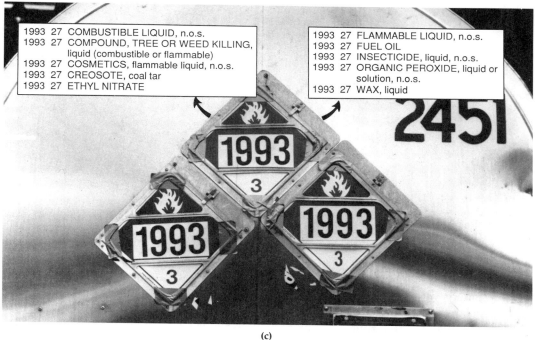

(c)

Figure 4–4 Using United Nations identification numbers, responders can identify specific chemicals and groups of chemicals. (a) By referring to U.S. Department of Transportation's *Emergency Response Guidebook,* methyl methacrylate can be identified by United Nations identification number 1247. (b) United Nations identification number 1086 refers to both monochloroethylene and vinyl chloride. (c) United Nations identification number 1993 alerts responders to the presence of a combustible liquid.

by individual chemicals and the quantities that are being transported. They must be used on motor vehicles, freight containers, and rail cars containing *any quantity* of the following materials that are regarded as the most dangerous of hazards:

- Class A explosives
- Class B explosives
- Class A poisons
- Water-reactive flammable solids
- Radioactive materials

For hazardous materials that are regarded as slightly less dangerous, placarding is required on motor vehicles, freight containers, and rail cars that contain 1,000 or more pounds. Materials for which these requirements apply include the following:

- Class B explosives
- Blasting agents
- Nonflammable gases
- Flammable gases
- Combustible liquids
- Flammable liquids
- Non-water–reactive flammable solids
- Oxidizers and organic peroxides
- Class B poisons
- Corrosives
- Irritating materials

These regulations are applied in a slightly different manner for shipments by air or water. In those cases, placards are required for any container larger than 640 cubic feet containing any quantity of the chemicals listed earlier.

Emergency use.   The purpose of placards and labels is to permit emergency responders to identify hazardous materials involved in accidents and emergencies rapidly so that appropriate protective responses can be taken. To assure the safety of responders, placards should be read from as far away as possible. For that purpose, emergency response teams should be equipped with binoculars that permit scene evaluation and placard interpretation from a safe distance.

Responders must also be able to interpret the meaning of placards. Placard colors, symbols, and their corresponding hazard classes should be learned by memory. UN chemical identification numbers can be interpreted by use of tables contained in the *Emergency Response Guidebook* published by DOT. This book is carried on nearly all emergency response vehicles in the United States. Once the UN number has been found on a placard, the *Guidebook* can be used to find a limited amount of generic emergency response information that is useful for initial response planning. In an emergency, responders should consult as many information texts and other resources as is practically possible to assure the correctness of response tactics and rescue plans. Additional resource documents are discussed in chapter 5.

Shipping Papers

When hazardous materials are being commercially transported, shipping papers are required that describe the material by name and identification number, its hazard class, quantity, and destination. These documents are usually in a standardized form and can provide useful information to emergency responders. Unfortunately, shipping papers are normally kept close to the hazardous materials and, therefore, obtaining them may be extremely difficult or not recommended during an emergency.

The types of shipping papers used, their location during transport, and the person responsible for them are presented in Table 4–4. An example of a bill of lading from a truck shipment is presented as Figure 4–5.

National Fire Protection Association (NFPA) Marking System

The NFPA has developed one of the most widely used emergency information systems for hazardous materials. Known as NFPA 704M, identification of the hazards of materials, this information scheme is illustrated in Figure 4–6. Information is provided that is relevant to the health, flammability, and reactivity risks of a chemical. The severity of each risk is ranked on a scale from 4 (greatest risk) to 0 (no risk). Each type of information is color coded: Health information is blue, flammability information is red, and reactivity information is yellow. The square diamond with points of blue, red, and yellow are often seen on chemical containers, and the color scheme has been widely adopted by industry as a means of designating the types of hazards associated with individual agents. The fourth corner at the bottom is white, and contains special information such as ''dangerous when wet'' or ''radioactive.''

Agricultural Chemical Warning System

Federal regulations require detailed information on the labels of agricultural chemicals such as pesticides, insecticides, and herbicides. Included in that information, along with identification of the product and use instructions, are state-

TABLE 4-4 SHIPPING PAPER IDENTIFICATION CHART*

Mode of transportation	Title of shipping paper	Location of shipping papers	Responsible person
Highway	Bill of lading	Cab of vehicle	Driver
Rail	Waybill Consist or wheel report	With Conductor or Engineer	Conductor
Water	Dangerous cargo Manifest	Wheelhouse or pipelike container on barge	Captain master
Air	Airbill with shippers certification for restricted articles	Cockpit[+]	Pilot

*Adapted from Charles Wright, National Fire Academy, *Recognizing and Identifying Hazardous Materials*, Emmitsburg, Md., 1985.
[+] Also may be found attached to outside of packages.

STRAIGHT BILL OF LADING — SHORT FORM — ORIGINAL — NOT NEGOTIABLE

Received, subject to the classifications and tariffs in effect on the date of the issue of the Bill of Lading.

Printed in U.S.A. NA 5241 4 PT. REV. 8-78 10-79

THE COMPANY FROM **AMERICAN CYANAMID COMPANY**

CONSIGNED TO & DESTINATION (SAME AS BELOW UNLESS OTHERWISE INDICATED)	CARRIER'S NO.	DATE SHIPPED
ANYTOWN Connecticut 06400		REQ SHP 02/01/89

MAIL OR STREET ADDRESS FOR PURPOSES OF NOTIFICATION ONLY

ANYTOWN
California
21555

SHIPPER'S NO. 366827

CONSIGNEE'S NO.	RECEIVED AT
011889	106 Anytown CT

RTE. CODE	ROUTE AND CARRIER	IF CHARGES ARE TO BE PREPAID WRITE OR STAMP HERE "PREPAID"
ACYX	AMER CYAN-COMP TRK	PREPAID

[illegible]

IN THE EVENT OF AN EMERGENCY INVOLVING THIS SHIPMENT, ENDANGERING LIFE, OR PROPERTY, CALL TOLL FREE — DAY OR NIGHT: 800 424-9300

IN HM COLUMN BELOW: - ENTER AN X TO DESIGNATE A HAZARDOUS MATERIAL

CAR INITIALS & NO.

NO. & KINDS PKGS.	FREIGHT CODE	HM	DESCRIPTION OF ARTICLES, SPECIAL MARKS AND EXCEPTIONS	CLASS OR RATE	* WEIGHT (SUBJ. TO COR.)
50 DRMS	002	X	RESIN SOLUTION FLAMMABLE LIQUID UN1866 RQ (XYLENE/FORMALDEHYDE) (PLASTIC MATERIAL, LIQUID) (MODIFIED MELAMINE RESIN IN MIXTURE OF BUTANOL & XYLENE) PRODUCT NO./NAME: 2618201 CYMEL 245-8		GROSS WT XXX 440 LBS
30 DRMS	002		PLASTIC MATERIAL, LIQUID (MODIFIED UREA RESIN IN ISOBUTANOL) PKG: 110 GALS OR LESS CAPACITY PRODUCT NO./NAME: 2653157 BEETLE 1032-10		XXX 440 LBS

Subject to Section 7 of conditions of applicable bill of lading, if this shipment is to be delivered to the consignee without recourse on the consignor, the consignor shall sign the following statement: The carrier shall not make delivery of this shipment without payment of freight and all other lawful charges.

(Signature of Consignor.)

Received $____ to apply in prepayment of the charges on the property described hereon.

Agent or Cashier

Per____ (The signature here acknowledges only the amount prepaid.)

Charges Advanced $____

* If the shipment moves between two ports by a carrier by water, the law requires that the bill of lading shall state whether it is carrier's or shipper's weight.

NOTE Where the rate is dependent on value, shippers are required to state specifically in writing the agreed or declared value of the property.

THE AGREED OR DECLARED VALUE OF THE PROPERTY IS HEREBY SPECIFICALLY STATED BY THE SHIPPER TO BE NOT EXCEEDING

50¢ PER POUND

This is to certify that the above-named materials are properly classified, described, packaged, marked and labeled, and are in proper condition for transportation according to the applicable regulations of the Department of Transportation.

AMERICAN CYANAMID COMPANY, Shipper,

Per SHIPPER SIGNS HERE

Agent____

Permanent Post Office Address of Shipper.

Per CARRIER SIGNS HERE

ORIGINAL B/L 4

Figure 4–5 An example of a bill of lading.

ments about hazard assessment and treatment of exposure victims. These labels are found on small containers as well as large shipping containers.

These labels are particularly useful for managing victims of exposure to these chemicals. When victims require transport and treatment in definitive centers of medical care, an uncontaminated label should be transported with the

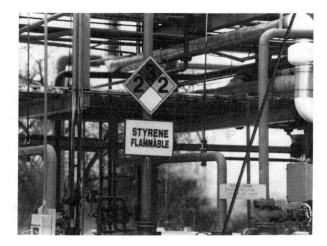

Figure 4–6 National Fire Protection Association 704 Marking System illustrating the effects of styrene.

patient to provide information for treatment. If that is not possible, the identity of the product, its components, and recommended medical treatment should be copied and passed along to the treatment center.

Material Safety Data Sheets (MSDS)

MSDS are information sheets that are used throughout industry as a means of identifying chemicals. MSDS contain summaries of the chemical and physical properties of chemicals, a brief overview of their health effects, and instruction for first aid of exposure victims. Federal regulations, developed by the OSHA, require that MSDS be provided to workers who are exposed to potentially hazardous chemicals during work.

    MSDS serve to identify chemicals and their properties and are widely used in industry. For that reason, emergency responders may be given these sheets when responding to emergencies at factories and other work sites. The emergency medical information that they contain is usually limited but accurate. A sample MSDS is presented as Figure 4–7.

SUMMARY

An effective and safe response to a hazardous materials accident cannot be carried out without appropriate information. Before any response or rescue is initiated, responders must determine whether hazardous materials are at the accident, what types of materials they are, and whether they are contributing to the emergency.

    Recognition of the presence of hazardous materials is based on suspicion. A rescuer may suspect the presence of hazards because of the location of the emergency or the presence of sensory clues.

ROHM AND HAAS COMPANY

CORPORATE PRODUCT INTEGRITY DEPARTMENT
INDEPENDENCE MALL WEST
PHILADELPHIA, PA 19105

EMERGENCY TELEPHONE
215-592-3000 (ROHM AND HAAS)
800-424-9300 (CHEMTREC)

HAZARD RATING
4=EXTREME
3=HIGH
2=MODERATE
1=SLIGHT
0=INSIGNIFICANT
··SEE SECTION IV

FIRE 1
REACTIVITY 1
TOXICITY 3
SPECIAL

MATERIAL SAFETY DATA SHEET — OSHA HAZARDOUS

LIST 10

MATERIAL	CODE	KEY	DOT HAZARD CLASS
AMMONIA ANHYDROUS - HOUSTON	70074	906563-7	NONFLAMMABLE GAS
	DATE ISSUED 11/26/86		

FORMULA	CHEMICAL NAME OR SYNONYMS
NH3	Ammonia gas

I — COMPOSITIONAL INFORMATION

	CAS Reg. No.	APPROX WT %	TWA/TLV
Ammonia	7664-41-7	100	R&H OSHA ACGIH 25 50 25 ppm

II — PHYSICAL PROPERTY INFORMATION

APPEARANCE - ODOR - pH.
Colorless gas, extremely pungent odor

VISCOSITY: NA

MELTING OR FREEZING POINT	BOILING POINT	VAPOR PRESSURE (mm Hg)	VAPOR DENSITY (AIR=1)
-78C/-108F	-33C/-28F	115 psi @ 20C/68F	0.6

SOLUBILITY IN WATER	PERCENT VOLATILE (BY WEIGHT)	SPECIFIC GRAVITY (WATER=1)	EVAPORATION RATE (BUTYL ACETATE=1)
Completely	100	0.618	>1

III — FIRE AND EXPLOSION HAZARD INFORMATION

FLASH POINT	AUTO IGNITION TEMPERATURE	LOWER EXPLOSION LIMIT (%)	UPPER EXPLOSION LIMIT (%)
NA	651C/1204F	16.0	25.0

EXTINGUISHING MEDIA: [X] FOAM [ ] "ALCOHOL" FOAM [ ] CO2 [X] DRY CHEMICAL [X] WATER SPRAY [ ] OTHER

SPECIAL FIRE FIGHTING PROCEDURES
Move containers promptly out of fire zone. If removal is impossible cool them with water spray. If escaping gas is burning, do not put out fire unless leak can be shut off immediately. Wear MSHA/NIOSH self-contained breathing apparatus and full protective clothing.

UNUSUAL FIRE AND EXPLOSION HAZARDS
Heated material can form explosive vapors with air. Fire produces toxic products: toxic ammonia fumes and oxides of nitrogen.

IV — HEALTH HAZARD INFORMATION

ROHM AND HAAS RECOMMENDED WORK PLACE EXPOSURE LIMITS
TWA--See SECTION I. STEL = 35 ppm

EFFECTS OF OVEREXPOSURE

Inhalation: Gas or vapor can cause severe irritation of nose and throat as well as nausea, coughing, chest pain and breathing difficulty.

Eye Contact: Severely irritating to eyes; possibly permanent injury

Skin Contact: Severely irritating to skin.

Ingestion: Substance will cause burning and severe swelling of the mouth, throat and abdomen.

EMERGENCY AND FIRST AID PROCEDURES
Inhalation: Material is extremely toxic: treatment must not be delayed! Move subject to fresh air. Give artificial respiration if unconscious. Get prompt medical attention.
Eye and Skin Contact: IMMEDIATELY flush eyes with running water for 15 minutes while forcibly holding eyelids open to permit water to irrigate all surfaces. Get under a safety shower. Remove clothing and flood skin with water for 30 minutes. Get prompt medical attention regardless of injury. Note: It is helpful to have someone other than the victim hold the eyes open.
Ingestion: If swallowed dilute by giving 2 glasses of water to drink. See a physician. Never give anything by mouth to an unconscious person.

Figure 4–7 A sample material safety data sheet form.

V — REACTIVITY INFORMATION

STABILITY	CONDITIONS TO AVOID
[X] STABLE [ ] UNSTABLE	Heat and flame.

HAZARDOUS DECOMPOSITION PRODUCTS
Fire may produce toxic ammonia fumes and oxides of nitrogen.

HAZARDOUS POLYMERIZATION	CONDITIONS TO AVOID
[ ] MAY OCCUR [X] WILL NOT OCCUR	NA

INCOMPATIBILITY (MATERIALS TO AVOID) [ ] WATER [X] OTHER
Silver, mercury, calcium, oxidizing gases, chlorine, bromine, iodine, hypochlorite and acids.

VI — SPILL OR LEAK PROCEDURE INFORMATION

STEPS TO BE TAKEN IN CASE MATERIAL IS RELEASED OR SPILLED
Eliminate ignition sources. Ventilate area. Avoid breathing gas. Wear protective clothing and respirator suitable for concentration encountered (MSHA/NIOSH-approved or equivalent). Use self-contained breathing apparatus (pressure-demand, MSHA/NIOSH-approved or equivalent) for large spills in confined area. Water spray may be effective in absorbing gas, but use around gas leaks only. Do not use on leaking containers or liquid spills. If liquid, dike and contain spill with inert material (e.g., sand, earth). Transfer liquid to containers for recovery or disposal and solid diking material to separate containers for disposal. Continued in Section VIII.

WASTE DISPOSAL METHODS
When discarded this material is a hazardous waste. Dilute with large quantities of water to a chemical sewer, in accordance with local, state and federal regulations.

VII — SPECIAL PROTECTION INFORMATION

VENTILATION TYPE
Mechanical local exhaust ventilation at point of contaminant release.

RESPIRATORY PROTECTION
Wear respirator (MSHA/NIOSH-approved or equivalent) suitable for concentrations encountered.

PROTECTIVE GLOVES	EYE PROTECTION
Impervious, rubber	Chemical splash goggles (ANSI Z-87.1 or approved equivalent)

OTHER PROTECTIVE EQUIPMENT
Eyewash facility, safety shower, protective clothing to prevent contact

VIII — STORAGE AND HANDLING INFORMATION

STORAGE TEMPERATURE MAX. MIN.	INDOOR	HEATED	REFRIGERATED	OUTDOOR

Store in a cool, well-ventilated area. Store away from excessive heat (e.g., steam pipes, radiators), from sources of ignition, and from reactive materials.

Spills (continued): Evacuate spill area if leak is large. Keep spills and cleaning run-offs out of municipal sewers and open bodies of water. Notify National Response Center if spill exceeds reportable quantity of 100 lbs./45 kg (40 CFR Part 302, "Superfund").

IX — TOXICITY INFORMATION

RTECS Reference B00875000:
Eye (rabbit): 100 mg severely irritating
Acute oral LD50 (rat): 350 mg/kg
Acute inhalation (mouse): 4837 ppm (1 hour)

X — MISCELLANEOUS INFORMATION

(1) Hercules Chemical Company, Wilmington, Delaware 19899, (302) 654-8900
(2) Herbert-Verkamp-Calvert Chemical Company, 4600 Dues Drive, Cincinnati, Ohio 45246, (513) 874-9267

NA = NOT APPLICABLE C = CEILING VALUE	KEY 906563-7	DATE OF ISSUE 11/26/86	SUPERSEDES 10/03/85

Figure 4–7 *(continued)*

Once hazardous materials have been recognized, efforts should be made to identify them specifically. This permits responders to take safety measures to avoid exposure, allows containment and mitigation efforts to be developed specifically for the actual hazard, and assures that the management of victims will be as appropriate as possible. Identification is based on an understanding of placards, labels, and other warning systems. Emergency responders should become familiar with these systems, and all emergency response vehicles should carry binoculars and reference books to facilitate identification.

REFERENCES

CARLSON, GENE P., ed., *HazMat Response Team Leak and Spill Guide.* Stillwater, Okla.: Fire Protection Publications, Oklahoma State University, 1984.

1987 Emergency Response Guidebook (4th ed.). Washington, D.C.: U.S. Department of Transportation, Materials Transportation Bureau, 1987.

IFSTA, *Hazardous Materials for First Responders* (1st ed.), ed. Gene P. Carlson. Stillwater, Okla.: Fire Protection Publications, Oklahoma State University, 1988.

ISMAN, WARREN E., and GENE P. CARLSON, *Hazardous Materials,* Encino, Calif.: Glencoe Publishing Co., 1980.

NATIONAL FIRE PROTECTION ASSOCIATION INC., *Fire Protection Guide on Hazardous Materials* (9th ed.), Quincy, Mass.: National Fire Protection Association, 1986.

NIOSH Pocket Guide to Chemical Hazards (5th ed.). The Division of Standards Development and Technology Transfer (DSDTT), NIOSH, Cincinnati, Ohio, 1985.

NOLL, GREGORY G., MICHAEL S. HILDEBRAND, and JAMES G. YVORRA, *Hazardous Materials Managing the Incident,* Office of Hazardous Materials Transportation, Research and Special Programs Administration, Stillwater, Okla.: Fire Protection Publications, Oklahoma State University, 1988.

HAZARDOUS MATERIALS
RISK ASSESSMENT
AND DATA GATHERING
CHAPTER 5

GOAL: On completion of this chapter the student will have an understanding of the more common sources of hazardous materials information.

OBJECTIVES:

Specifically, the student will be able to

- Name the general categories of resources available to responders about hazardous materials
- Name at least six emergency response guidebooks that are available to emergency responders
- Name at least three electronic data base systems that are available to emergency responders
- Name at least six 24-hour telephone access systems that are available to emergency responders
- Describe the Hazards Communication Standard
- Describe the information provided on material safety data sheets
- Describe the major requirements of the Superfund Amendments and Reauthorization Act of 1986

OVERVIEW

To assess the risks posed by hazardous materials accidents and to develop adequate response and rescue plans, emergency responders need accurate information about the hazards with which they must deal. In chapter 4, some of these informational concerns were discussed, particularly the recognition of hazardous materials at an accident and the identification of those materials. Recognition and identification are critical first steps in gathering data about a hazardous materials accident. Such information allows responders to take appropriate safety precautions and begin rescue planning.

In most cases, however, identification of the hazardous materials does not provide enough information to develop a comprehensive response plan. One problem is that so many hazardous materials exist and each can cause so many potential forms of harm that few persons are able to remember much about any one of them. Emergency responders will almost always need to research the chemicals involved at an accident to be certain that they understand the specific dangers that are posed and the specific care required by victims.

In this chapter, some of the more common sources of hazardous materials information will be reviewed that are generally available to emergency responders. These data sources include the following:

- Books and printed materials
- Electronic data bases
- Telephone information services
- Right-to-know forms

It is not likely that response personnel will know or use all of these information sources. Some familiarity with them, however, will be helpful. Response personnel should practice using those data sources that will most often be available to them at an emergency. In this way, responders can be confident that they know how and when to use each. Emergency response services should maintain a portable library or electronic data retrieval system to access needed data sources readily at the accident scene. In general, rescuers should research hazardous materials in three or more different sources of information.

BOOKS AND PRINTED MATERIALS

Many emergency response guidebooks are available that contain information on hazardous materials. A selected group are described subsequently. Most are primarily concerned with issues of flammability and reactivity. Some are useful for identification of chemicals. Most provide little information on the health effects of acute exposures or the health care needs of acute exposure victims. As a result, most of these information sources are of greater value to fire service responders than EMS personnel.

The flammability and reactivity information contained in these response guidebooks generally include summaries of a hazardous material's physical and chemical properties such as the following:

- Melting and boiling points
- Vapor pressure and density
- Solubility
- Flash point
- Flammable (explosive) range
- Autoignition (ignition) temperature
- Chemical incompatibilities

Most of the guidebooks include information on the selection of personal protective equipment. Included are the types of respirators and protective clothing needed to enter a contaminated environment. Others include specific descriptions of approved techniques for containing spills and extinguishing fires.

In most cases, the health-related data included are limited to statements about the organ systems likely to be affected by exposure and first aid for victims. Such information may be useful for untrained rescuers, but does not provide proper guidance for EMS and medical personnel. Fortunately, as noted subsequently, a few good sources of emergency medical information are available.

EMS organizations must devote extra effort to assemble the kinds of health care information needed at a hazardous materials emergency. Emergency medical responders should not assume that information sources that are adequate for fire service personnel will also provide the data and guidelines necessary for health care emergencies.

Listed subsequently and in the following sections are some commonly used emergency response guidebooks and other sources of emergency response information. Particular emphasis has been placed on those that provide information on the health effects of exposure. It is likely that other good references and information sources that have not been included here are available. Emergency responders are encouraged to examine as many information sources as possible before determining those that will be used on a regular basis.

1987 Emergency Response Guidebook.   *Office of Hazardous Materials Transportation, Research and Special Programs Administration, Washington, D.C.: U.S. Department of Transportation, 1987.*

This guidebook was discussed earlier in chapter 4. It is useful for identifying hazardous materials involved in transportation accidents. By means of the UN identification number, it is possible to determine a chemical's identity quickly and establish an initial action plan. This book should be carried in all fire vehicles, police cars, and ambulances. It does not provide useful technical or health care information. A sample of the index and guide pages are presented in Figure 5–1.

ID No.	Guide No.	Name of Material	ID No.	Guide No.	Name of Material
0004	46	AMMONIUM PICRATE, dry or wetted with less than 10% water	1015	12	CARBON DIOXIDE-NITROUS OXIDE MIXTURE
0222	46	AMMONIUM NITRATE FERTI-LIZER, with not more likely 2% of combustible material	1016	18	CARBON MONOXIDE
			1017	20	**CHLORINE ***
0223	46	AMMONIUM NITRATE FERTI-LIZER, which is more likely to explode than UN0222	1018	12	CHLORODIFLUOROMETHANE
			1020	12	CHLOROPENT.AFLUORO-ETHANE
0357	46	SUBSTANCES, EXPLOSIVE	1021	12	CHLOROTETRAFLUORO-ETHANE
0358	46	SUBSTANCES, EXPLOSIVE	1022	12	CHLOROTRIFLUOROMETHANE
0359	46	SUBSTANCES, EXPLOSIVE	1022	12	TRIFLUOROCHLORO-METHANE
0402	46	AMMONIUM PERCHLORATE, average particle size of less than 45 microns	1023	18	COAL GAS
			1026	18	CYANOGEN
1001	17	ACETYLENE	1026	18	**CYANOGEN, liquefied ***
1001	17	ACETYLENE, dissolved	1027	22	CYCLOPROPANE
1002	12	AIR, compressed	1027	22	CYCLOPROPANE, liquefied
1003	23	AIR, refrigerated liquid (cryogenic liquid)	1028	12	DICHLORODIFLUOROMETHANE
			1029	12	DICHLOROFLUOROMETHANE
1005	15	**AMMONIA ***	1029	12	DICHLOROMONOFLUORO-METHANE
1005	15	**AMMONIA, ANHYDROUS, liquefied ***	1030	22	DIFLUOROETHANE
1005	15	**ANHYDROUS AMMONIA ***	1032	19	**DIMETHYLAMINE, anhydrous ***
1006	12	ARGON, compressed	1033	22	DIMETHYL ETHER
1008	15	**BORON TRIFLUORIDE ***	1035	22	ETHANE, compressed
1009	12	BROMOTRIFLUOROMETHANE	1036	68	ETHYLAMINE
1010	17	BUTADIENE, inhibited	1036	68	MONOETHYLAMINE
1011	22	BUTANE or BUTANE MIXTURE	1037	27	ETHYL CHLORIDE
1012	22	BUTENE	1038	22	ETHYLENE, cryogenic liquid
1012	22	BUTYLENE	1038	22	ETHYLENE, liquid (refrigerated)
1013	21	CARBON DIOXIDE	1039	26	ETHYL METHYL ETHER
1014	14	CARBON DIOXIDE-OXYGEN MIXTURE	1039	26	METHYL ETHYL ETHER

Figure 5–1 *1987 Emergency Response Guidebook* index page for ammonia showing United Nations identification and guide numbers for further reference.

GUIDE 15

POTENTIAL HAZARDS

HEALTH HAZARDS
Poisonous; may be fatal if inhaled or absorbed through skin.
Contact may cause burns to skin and eyes.
Contact with liquid may cause frostbite.
Runoff from fire control or dilution water may cause pollution.

FIRE OR EXPLOSION
Some of these materials may burn, but none of them ignites readily.
Cylinder may explode in heat of fire.

EMERGENCY ACTION

Keep unnecessary people away; isolate hazard area and deny entry.
Stay upwind, out of low areas, and ventilate closed spaces before entering.
Self-contained breathing apparatus (SCBA) and structural firefighter's protective
   clothing will provide limited protection for short-term exposure to these materials.
Fully-encapsulated protective clothing should be worn for spills and leaks with no
   fire.
Evacuate the leak or spill area immediately for at least 50 feet in all directions. (See
   the Table of Initial Evacuation Distances in the back of this book. If you find the
   Name of Material there, call for help to perform the recommended evacuation.)
CALL CHEMTREC AT 1-800-424-9300 AS SOON AS POSSIBLE, especially if there is
   no local hazardous materials team available.

FIRE
Small Fires: Dry chemical, CO2 or Halon.
Large Fires: Water spray, fog or standard foam is recommended.
Do not get water inside container.
Move container from fire area if you can do it without risk.
Cool containers that are exposed to flames with water from the side until well after
   fire is out. Stay away from ends of tanks.
Isolate area until gas has dispersed.

SPILL OR LEAK
Stop leak if you can do it without risk.
Use water spray to reduce vapor; **do not** put water directly on leak or spill area.
Small Spills: Flush area with flooding amounts of water.
Large Spills: Dike far ahead of liquid spill for later disposal.
Do not get water inside container.
Isolate area until gas has dispersed.

FIRST AID
Move victim to fresh air and call emergency medical care; if not breathing, give ar-
   tificial respiration; if breathing is difficult, give oxygen.
Remove and isolate contaminated clothing and shoes at the site.
In case of contact with material, immediately flush skin or eyes with running water
   for at least 15 minutes.
Keep victim quiet and maintain normal body temperature.
Effects may be delayed; keep victim under observation.

Figure 5–1 (*continued*) *1987 Emergency Response Guidebook* guide page for ammonia showing health hazards, fire or explosion hazards, and recommended
emergency action.

NIOSH Pocket Guide to Chemical Hazards. *The Division of Standards Development and Technology Transfer, NIOSH, Cincinnati, Ohio, U.S. Department of Health and Human Services, 1985.*

This pocket-sized guidebook contains an assortment of technical information about individual chemicals. It is a useful source of information on physical and chemical properties, some health exposure limits (particularly PEL and IDLH values), and use of personal protective equipment. Brief summaries of health effects and first-aid procedures are included. A sample guidebook page is presented in Figure 5–2.

Sax, N. I., and R. J. Lewis, Dangerous Properties of Industrial Materials. *New York: Van Nostrand Reinhold Co., 1989.*

This comprehensive work contains extensive data presented in table form, which include physical and chemical properties, flammability and reactivity risks, health exposure limits, guidelines for personal protective equipment, and simple first-aid directions. A sample page is presented in Figure 5–3.

Meyer, E., Chemistry of Hazardous Materials. *Englewood Cliffs, N.J.: Brady Books, 1989.*

This comprehensive work is a textbook of chemistry that specifically discusses substances that act as hazardous materials. The toxicity of many com-

Chemical Name, Formula, CAS, RTECS, and DOT UN or NA and Guide Numbers	Synonyms	Exposure Limits	IDLH Level	Physical Description	Chemical and Physical Properties		Incompatibilities	Measurement Method (See Tables 1a and 1b)
Ammonia NH₃ 7664-41-7 BO0875000 1005 15	Anhydrous ammonia	50 ppm (35 mg/m³) (NIOSH) 50 ppm 5-min ceil (35 mg/m³) (ACGIH) 25 ppm	500 ppm	Colorless gas with a penetrating, pungent, suffocating odor; can be a liquid when under pressure	MW: 17 BP: -28°F Sol: 51% Fl.P: None IP: 10.15 eV	VP: >1 atm MP: -108°F UEL: 25% LEL: 16%	Strong oxidizers, calcium, hypochlorite bleaches, gold, mercury, silver, halogens	SiO + H₂SO₄; ISE; Set 6
Ammonium sulfamate NH₂SO₃NH₄ 7773-06-0 WO6125000 9089 31	Ammate herbicide	15 mg/m³ (ACGIH) 10 mg/m³	5000 mg/m³	Colorless, odorless solid	MW: 114 BP: 392°F Sol: 200% Not combustible	VP: ≅0 mm MP: 268°F	Strong oxidizers, hot water	NIOSH 79-141
n-Amyl acetate CH₃COOC₅H₁₁ 628-63-7 AJ1925000 1104 26	1-Pentanol acetate, n-Amyl acetate (mixed isomers)	100 ppm (525 mg/m³)	4000 ppm	Colorless liquid with a banana oil odor	MW: 130 BP: 295°F Sol: 0.2% Fl.P: 77°F	VP: 4 mm MP: -95°F UEL: 7.5% LEL: 1.1%	Nitrates; strong oxidizers, alkalies, and acids	Char; CS₂; GC; III
sec-Amyl acetate C₇H₁₄O₂ 626-38-0 AJ2100000 1104 26	2-Pentanol acetate	125 ppm (650 mg/m³)	9000 ppm	Clear, colorless liquid with a fruity odor	MW: 130 BP: 273°F Sol: 0.2% Fl.P: 89°F	VP: 7 mm MP: -148°F UEL: ? LEL: 1% (est)	Nitrates; strong oxidizers, alkalies, and acids	Char; CS₂; GC; III

Figure 5–2 *NIOSH Pocket Guide to Chemical Hazards* sample pages for ammonia.

Personal Protection and Sanitation (See Table 2)	Respirator Selection Upper Limit Devices Recommended (See Table 3)	Health Hazards			
		Route	Symptoms (See Table 4)	First Aid (See Table 5)	Target Organs

Clothing: > 10% AP/≤ 10% RP
Goggles: > 10% AP/≤ RP
Wash: > 10% imm con/
     ≤ 10% pro wet
Change: N.A.
Remove: Non-imp con > 10% imm/
     ≤ 10%
Provide: Eyewash and drench
     > 10%
	NIOSH
	300 ppm: CCRS*
	500 ppm: SA*:PAPRS*
	GMFS/SCBA*
	Ω: SCBAF:PD,PP/
	SAF:PD,PP:ASCBA
	Escape: GMFS/SCBAE
		Inh
		Ing
		Con
			Eye, nose, throat irrit;
			dysp; bronspas; chest
			pain; pulm edema; pink
			frothy sputum; skin
			burns; vesic
				Eye: Irr immed
				Skin: Water flush immed
				Breath: Art resp
				Swallow: Medical attention
				    immed
					Resp sys,
					eyes

Clothing: N.A. Goggles: N.A. Wash: N.A. Change: N.A. Remove: N.A.	ACGIH 50 mg/m³: DM 100 mg/m³:DMXSQ/SA 250 mg/m³: PAPRDM/SA:CF 500 mg/m³: HiEF/PAPRTHiE/ SAT:CF/SCBAF/SAF 5000 mg/m³: SA:PD,PP Ω: SCBAF:PD,PP/ SAF:PD,PP:ASCBA Escape: HiEF/SCBAE	Inh Ing Con	None known in humans	Eye: Irr immed Skin: Soap wash promptly Breath: Art resp Swallow: Medical attention immed	None known

Clothing: Repeat prolong
Goggles: Reason prob
Wash: Promptly upon wet
Change: N.A.
Remove: Any wet immed (flamm)
	OSHA
	1000 ppm: PAPROV*/CCROV*
	SA*/SCBA*
	2500 ppm: SA:CF*
	4000 ppm: GMFOV/SCBAF/SAF
	Ω: SCBAF:PD,PP/
	SAF:PD,PP:ASCBA
	Escape: GMFOV/SCBAE
		Ihn
		Ing
		Con
			Irrit eyes, nose; narcosis;
			derm
				Eye: Irr immed
				Skin: Water flush
				    promptly
				Breath: Art resp
				Swallow: Medical attention
				    immed
					Eyes, skin, resp
					sys

Clothing: Repeat prolong
Goggles: Reason prob
Wash: Promptly upon wet
Change: N.A.
Remove: Any wet immed (flamm)
	OSHA
	1000 ppm: PAPROV*/CCROV*
	1250 ppm: SA*/SCBA*
	3125 ppm: SA:CF*
	6250 ppm: GMFOV/SCBAF/SAF
	9000 ppm: SAF:PD,PP
	Ω: SCBAF:PD,PP/
	SAF:PD,PP:ASCBA
	Escape: GMFOV/SCBAE
		Inh
		Ing
		Con
			Irrit eyes, nose; narcosis;
			derm
				Eye: Irr immed
				Skin: Water flush
				    promptly
				Breath: Art resp
				Swallow: Medical attention
				    immed
					Resp sys, eyes,
					skin

sec-Amyl acetate

Figure 5–2 (*continued*)

pounds are discussed briefly, but no treatment protocols or clinical guidelines are provided.

Bronstein, A. C., P. L. Currance, *Emergency Care for Hazardous Materials Exposure.* St. Louis: The C. V. Mosby Company, 1988.

This guidebook is patterned after the *DOT Emergency Response Guidebook* described earlier. Chemicals are listed in an index which then refers users to one of eighty-two treatment guidelines. It contains no information on exposure limits, but useful management protocols for EMS personnel and brief summaries of health effects are given. A sample guideline is presented in Figure 5–4.

Proctor, N. H., J. P. Hughes, M. L. Fischman, *Chemical Hazards of the Workplace.* Philadelphia: J. B. Lippincott, 1988.

A comprehensive occupational medicine text that devotes one to four pages to many toxic industrial chemicals. Good discussions of toxicology, clinical symptoms and signs, and diagnosis of exposure to individual chemicals. The previous edition of this book (1978) also contained useful information on treatment but that is no longer included. This textbook is too advanced for EMS personnel, but it is useful for emergency departments and medical control physicians. A sample entry is presented in Figure 5–5.

AMY500
AMMONIA   *HR: 3*
CAS: 7664-41-7
DOT: 1005   NIOSH: BO 0875000
mf: H_3N mw: 17.04

PROP: Colorless gas, extremely pungent odor, liquefied by compression. Mp: $-77.7°$, bp: $-33.35°$, lel: 16%, uel: 25%, d: 0.771 g/liter @ 0°, 0.817 g/liter @ $-79°$, autoign temp: 1204°F, vap press: 10 atm @ 25.7°, vap d: 0.6. Very sol in water, moderately sol in alc.

SYNS:
AMMONIA ANHYDROUS	AMMONIAK (GERMAN)
AMMONIAC (FRENCH)	AMONIAK (POLISH)
AMMONIACA (ITALIAN)	SPIRIT OF HARTSHORN
AMMONIA GAS	

TOXICITY DATA: CODEN:

mmo-esc 1500 ppm/3H	AMNTA4 85,119,51
cyt-rat-ihl 19800 µg/m³/16W	BZARAZ 27,102,74
ihl-hmn LCLo: 30000 ppm/5M	TJSGA8 45,458,67
ihl-hmn TCLo: 20 ppm: IRR	AGGHAR 13,528,55
unk-man LDLo: 132 mg/kg	85DCAI 2,73,70
orl-rat LD50: 350 mg/kg	PHIT**
ihl-rat LCLo: 2000 ppm/4H	JIHTAB 31,343,49
ihl-mus LD50: 4837 ppm/1H	NTIS** PB214-270
ihl-cat LCLo: 7000 ppm/1H	JIHTAB 26,29,44
ihl-cat TCLo: 1000 ppm/10M	AEHLAU 35,6,80
ihl-rbt LCLo: 7000 ppm/1H	JIHTAB 26,29,44
ihl-mam LCLo: 5000 ppm/5M	AEPPAE 138,65,28

EPA Extremely Hazardous Substances List. Community Right To Know List. Reported in EPA TSCA Inventory.

OSHA PEL: TWA 50 ppm
ACGIH TLV: TWA 25 ppm; STEL 35 ppm
DFG MAK: 50 ppm (35 mg/m³)
NIOSH REL: CL 50 ppm

DOT Classification: Nonflammable Gas, Label: Nonflammable Gas

THR: A human poison by an unspecified route. Poison experimentally by inhalation, ingestion, and possibly other routes. An eye, mucous membrane, and systemic irritant by inhalation. Mutagenic data. A common air contaminant. Difficult to ignite. Explosion hazard when exposed to flame or in a fire. NH_3 + air in a fire can detonate. Potentially violent or explosive reactions on contact with interhalogens (e.g., bromine pentafluoride; chlorine trifluoride); 1,2-dichloroethane (with liquid NH_3); boron halides; chloroformamidnium nitrate; ethylene oxide (polymerization reaction); magnesium perchlorate; nitrogen trichloride; oxygen + platinum; or strong oxidants (e.g., potassium chlorate; nitryl chloride; chromyl chloride; dichlorine oxide; chromium trioxide; trioxygen difluoride; nitric acid; hydrogen peroxide; tetramethylammonium amide; thiocarbonyl azide thiocyanate; sulfinyl chloride; thiotriazyl chloride; ammonium peroxodisulfate; fluorine; nitrogen oxide; dinitrogen tetraoxide; and liquid oxygen). Forms sensitive explosive mixtures with air + hydrocarbons; 1-chloro-2,4-dinitrobenzene; 2-,or 4-chloronitrobenzene (above 160°C/30 bar); ethanol + silver nitrate; germanium derivatives; stibine; and chlorine. Reaction with silver chloride; silver nitrate; silver azide; and silver oxide form the explosive silver nitride. Reactions with chlorine azide; bromine; iodine; iodine + potassium; heavy metals and their compounds (e.g. gold(III) chloride; mercury; and potassium thallium amide ammoniate); tellurium halides (e.g., tellurium tetrabromide; and tellurium tetrachloride)and pentaborane(9) give explosive products. Incompatible in contact with Ag; acetaldehyde; acrolein; B; BI_3; halogens; $HClO_3$; ClO; chlorites; chlorosilane; (ethylene dichloride + liquid ammonia); Au; hexachloromelamine; (hydrazine + alkali metals); HBr; HOCl; $Mg(ClO_4)_2$; N_2O_4; NCl_3; NF_3; OF_2; P_2O_5; P_2O_3; picric acid; (K + AsH_3); (K + PH_3); (K + $NaNO_2$); potassium ferricyanide; potassium mercuric cyanide; (Na + CO); Sb; S; SCl_2; tellurium hydropentachloride; trichloromelamine; NO_2Cl; SbH_3; tetramethylammonium amide; $SOCl_2$; thiotrithiazylchloride. Incandescent reaction when heated with calcium. Emits toxic fumes of NH_3 and NO_x when exposed to heat. Stop flow of gas to fight fire. For further information, see Vol. 3, No. 3 of *DPIM Report*.

AMZ125   *HR: 2*
2-AMMONIOTHIAZOLE NITRATE
CAS: 57530-25-3
mf: $C_3H_5N_3O_3S$ mw: 163.15

THR: Explosive decomposition at 142°C. Upon decomposition it emits toxic fumes of SO_x and NO_x.

ANA000   *HR: 3*
AMMONIUM ACETATE
CAS: 631-61-8
DOT: 9079   NIOSH: AF 3675000
mf: $C_2H_4O_2 \cdot H_3N$ mw: 77.10

PROP: Crystals. Mp: 114°, d: 1.07.

SYN: ACETIC ACID, AMMONIUM SALT

TOXICITY DATA: CODEN:

ivn-mus LD50: 386 mg/kg	MEIEDD 10,74,83
ipr-rat LD50: 632 mg/kg	ABBIA4 64,342,56
ivn-mus LD50: 98 mg/kg	12VXA5 8,65,68
ipr-ckn LDLo: 1735 mg/kg	BIJOAK 106,699,68

Reported in EPA TSCA Inventory.

DOT Classification: ORM-E; Label: None

THR: Poison by intravenous route. Moderately toxic by intraperitoneal routes. When heated to decomposition it emits toxic fumes of NO_x and NH_3. For further information, see Vol. 2, No. 3 of *DPIM Report*.

ANA250   *HR: 3*
AMMONIUM aci-NITROMETHANE
mf: $CH_7O_2N_2$ mw: 79.1

Figure 5–3 *Dangerous Properties of Industrial Materials* sample page for ammonia. (Reprinted with permission from Van Nostrand Reinhold, New York, N.Y.).

NUMERICAL INDEX

UN #	CHEMICAL NAME	GUIDELINE #
0072	Cyclonite	54
0076	2,4, Dinitrophenol	38
0154	Picric Acid	1,38 & 59
0208	Tetryl	1
0209	Trinitrotoluene	19
0214	Trinitrobenzene	19
1001	Acetylene	72
1005	Ammonia, Anhydrous, Liquified	18
1006	Argon, Compressed	79
1008	Boron Trifluoride	14
1009	Bromotrifluoromethane	72
1009	Monobromotrifluoromethane	72
1009	Trifluorobromomethane	3
1010	1,3, Butadiene	72
1011	n-Butane	72
1012	Butylene	16
1013	Carbon Dioxide	79
1015	Carbon Dioxide-Nitrous Oxide Mixture	79
1016	Carbon Monoxide	29
1017	Chlorine	74
1018	Chlorodifluoromethane	3
1020	Chloropentafluoroethane	41
1020	Monochloropentafluoroethane	72
1021	Chlorotetrafluoroethane	41
1021	Monochlorotetrafluoroethane	72
1022	Chlorotrifluoromethane	41
1022	Monochlorotrifluoromethane	72
1026	Cyanogen	33
1027	Cyclopropane	72
1028	Dichlorodifluoromethane	3

Figure 5–4 Sample index page for ammonia showing United Nations identification and guide numbers for further reference. (Reproduced with permission from *Emergency Care for Hazardous Materials Exposure*, A. C. Bronstein and P. L. Currance, St. Louis, 1988, The C. V. Mosby Company.)

Morgan, D. P., Recognition and Management of Pesticide Poisonings. Washington, D.C.: U.S. Environmental Protection Agency, 1982.

This brief yet comprehensive discussion of pesticide poisonings includes discussions of the mechanisms of injury, clinical effects, and management strategies for exposure victims. This unique and easy-to-use reference contains more information than most EMS personnel would want or need, but it is useful for emergency departments and medical control physicians.

GUIDELINE 18

SUBSTANCE IDENTIFICATION: Found as ammonia in solution and as a colorless, anhydrous gas. Used as cleaning agents, fertilizers, and industrial refrigerants.

ROUTES OF EXPOSURE:

Skin and eye contact

Inhalation

Ingestion

LIFE THREAT: Acute pulmonary edema and hypotension.

SIGNS & SYMPTOMS BY SYSTEM:

Cardiovascular—Ventricular arrhythmias and hypotension.

Respiratory—Acute pulmonary edema, bronchospasm, stridor, cough, dyspnea, and chest pain. Respiratory tract irritation with possible laryngeal edema.

CNS—Stupor, lethargy, and coma. Seizures may be present.

Gastrointestinal—G.I. bleeding due to liquification necrosis of the G.I. tract.

Eye—Chemical conjunctivitis with vapors, necrosis, and blindness with liquids and anhydrous gas exposures.

Skin—Full and partial thickness burns with skin contact.

Other—Respiratory damage can be severe with potential fatal results. Respiratory symptoms may be delayed.

DECONTAMINATION:

- Wear positive pressure self-contained breathing apparatus and special protective equipment.
- Delay entry until equipment is available.
- Remove patient from contaminated area.
- Gently blot, with absorbent material, any excess liquids that are present.
- Rinse patient with water and remove all clothing, jewelry, and shoes.
- Wash patient with Tincture of Green Soap and large quantities of water.
- Refer to decontamination protocol in Section III.

BASIC TREATMENT:

- Assist ventilations as needed.
- Administer oxygen by nonrebreather mask at 6 to 12 L/min.
- Monitor for signs of pulmonary edema and treat as necessary (refer to pulmonary edema protocol in Section III).
- Monitor for shock and treat as necessary (refer to shock protocol in Section III).
- Anticipate seizures and treat as necessary (refer to seizure protocol in Section III).
- Flush eye immediately with available water for eye contamination. In adults, if lid and globe are intact and without edema, eye irrigation lens may be used. Do not force lens; if unable to insert easily, do not use. For children, and if unable to use irrigation lens in adults, flush eyes using large bore IV tubing. Irrigate each eye with a minimum of 1000 ccs of normal saline (refer to eye irrigation protocol in Section III).
- Administer 4 to 8 oz of water for dilution if product was ingested and the patient can swallow, has a good gag reflex, and no drooling.
- Do not use emetics.

Figure 5–4 (continued) Sample guide page for ammonia showing recommended care instructions. (*Emergency Care for Hazardous Materials Exposure*, A. C. Bronstein and P. L. Currance, St. Louis, 1988, The C. V. Mosby Company; reproduced with permission.)

Lefèvre, M. J., First Aid Manual for Chemical Accidents. *New York: Van Nostrand Reinhold Co., 1980.*

This guidebook is similar in design to the *DOT Emergency Response Guidebook*. Chemicals are listed in an index that then refers users to the appropriate pages of five separate sections dealing with symptoms of poisoning and first aid

ADVANCED TREATMENT:

- Consider orotracheal or nasotracheal intubation for airway control if signs of upper airway obstruction are present in the unconscious or severe pulmonary edema patient.
- Use positive pressure ventilation techniques; they may be beneficial.
- Monitor cardiac rhythm and treat arrhythmias as necessary (refer to cardiac protocol in Section III),·
- Start an IV with LR TKO.
- Consider drug therapy for pulmonary edema (refer to pulmonary edema protocol in Section III).
- Use pneumatic antishock garment and fluid resuscitation cautiously to treat hypotension with signs of hypovolemia and consider vasopressors if hypotensive with a normal fluid volume. Watch for signs of fluid overload (refer to shock protocol in Section III).
- Treat seizures with diazepam (Valium®). DOSAGE: 2 to 10 mg in 2 mg increments slow IV push (refer to diazepam protocol in Section IV).
- Use proparacaine hydrochloride to assist eye irrigation (refer to proparacaine hydrochloride protocol in Section IV).

Figure 5–4   (*continued*)

for inhalation, ingestion, and skin and eye contact. Treatment protocols are less advanced than those in *Emergency Care for Hazardous Materials Exposure*. Symptoms are considered, but long-term effects and exposure limits are not.

Stutz, D. R., S. J. Janusz, Hazardous Materials Injuries.   Beltsville, Md.: Bradford Communications, 1988.

This guidebook is also similar to the *DOT Emergency Response Guidebook*. More than three thousand chemicals are listed in an index that refers readers to one of ninety-eight treatment protocols. Protocols are similar to those in *Emergency Care for Hazardous Materials Exposure*. A summary of symptoms and health effects is provided, but information on exposure limits is not. The protocols and other related information is also available as a computer data base (see later). Discussions of decontamination procedures and personal protective equipment are contained in appendixes. A sample entry is provided in Figure 5–6.

Medical First Aid Guide for Use in Accidents Involving Dangerous Goods.   Geneva: International Maritime Organization, 1985.

This guidebook is a supplement to the *International Medical Guide for Ships*. It is divided into four principal sections: an overview of "first aid" including cardiopulmonary resuscitation; a review of complications from hazardous materials exposure; a summary of emergency treatment for exposure victims; and more than eighty tables that present summaries of the clinical effects of groups of hazardous materials and reference to emergency treatments protocols. Treatment protocols·are less advanced than those in *Emergency Care for Hazardous Materials Exposure*. Long-term effects and exposure limits are not considered.

AMMONIA
CAS: 7664-41-7
NH₃   1987 TLV = 25 ppm

Synonyms: Ammonia gas

Physical Form. Colorless gas

Uses. Refrigeration; petroleum refining; blueprint machines; manufacture of fertilizers, nitric acid, explosives, plastics, and other chemicals

Exposure. Inhalation

Toxicology. Ammonia is a severe irritant of the eyes, respiratory tract, and skin.

Exposure to and inhalation of concentrations of 2500 to 6500 ppm, as might result from accidents with liquid anhydrous ammonia, causes severe corneal irritation, dyspnea, bronchospasm, chest pain, and pulmonary edema, which may be fatal. Upper airway obstruction from laryngopharyngeal edema and desquamation of mucous membranes may occur early in the course and require endotracheal intubation or tracheostomy.[1-3] Case reports have documented chronic airway hyperreactivity and asthma, with associated obstructive pulmonary function changes following massive ammonia exposures.[3,4]

In a human experimental study that exposed 10 subjects to various vapor concentrations for 5 minutes, 134 ppm caused irritation of the eyes, nose, and throat in most subjects and 1 person complained of chest irritation; at 72 ppm, several subjects reported the same symptoms; at 50 ppm, 2 reported nasal dryness; and, at 32 ppm, only 1 person reported nasal dryness.[2] Surveys of workers have generally found that the maximal concentration not resulting in significant complaints is 20 to 25 ppm.[2]

Tolerance to usually irritating concentrations of ammonia may be acquired by adaptation, a phenomenon frequently observed among workers who became inured to the effects of exposure; no data are available on concentrations that are irritating to workers who are regularly exposed to ammonia and who presumably have a higher irritation threshold.

Liquid anhydrous ammonia in contact with the eyes may cause serious injury to the cornea and deeper structures and sometimes blindness; on the skin, it causes first- and second-degree burns, which are often severe and, if extensive, may be fatal. Vapor concentrations of 10,000 ppm are mildly irritating to the moist skin, whereas 30,000 ppm or greater cause a stinging sensation and may produce skin burns and vesiculation.[2] With skin and mucous membrane contact, burns occur in three ways: (1) cryogenic (from the liquid ammonia), (2) thermal (from the exothermic dissociation of ammonium hydroxide), and (3) chemical (alkaline).[3]

REFERENCES

1. Department of Labor: Exposure to ammonia, proposed standard. Federal Register 40:54684–54693, 1975
2. National Institute for Occupational Safety and Health, US Department of Health, Education and Welfare: Criteria for a Recommended Standard . . . Occupational Exposure to Ammonia. DHEW (NIOSH) Pub No 74–136. Washington, DC, US Government Printing Office, 1974
3. Arwood R, Hammond J, Ward G: Ammonia inhalation. Trauma 25(5):444–447, 1985
4. Flury K, Dines D, Rodarto J, Rodgers R: Airway obstruction due to inhalation of ammonia. Mayo Clin Proc 58:389–393, 1983

Figure 5–5 *Chemical Hazards of the Workplace* sample entry for ammonia. (Proctor N.H., Hughes J. P.: *Chemical Hazards of the Workplace,* J. P. Lippincott Co., 1988; reproduced with permission.)

NUMERICAL INDEX		
CHEMICAL NAME	UN/NA	PROTOCOL
Ammonium Picrate, dry or wetted with less than 10% water	0004	55
Trinitrophenol, dry or wetted, with less than 30% water by weight	0154	71
Ammonium Nitrate Fertilizer, with not more likely 2% of combustible material	0222	72
Ammonium Nitrate Fertilizer, which is more likely to explode than UN0222	0223	72
Substances, Explosive	0357	41
Substances, Explosive	0358	41
Substances, Explosive	0359	41
Ammonium Perchlorate, average particle size	0402	28
Acetylene	1001	48
Acetylene, dissolved	1001	48
Air, compressed	1002	66
Air, refrigerated liquid (cryogenic liquid)	1003	66
Ammonia	1005	9
Ammonia Anhydrous, Liquified	1005	9
Anhydrous Ammonia	1005	6
Argon, Compressed	1006	14
Boron Trifluoride	1008	18
Bromotrifluoromethane	1009	50
Monobromotrifluoromethane	1009	50
Butadiene, Inhibited	1010	48
Butane or Butane Mixture	1011	14
Butene	1012	14
Butylene	1012	48
Carbon Dioxide	1013	14
Carbon Dioxide-Oxygen Mixture	1014	66
Carbon Dioxide-Nitrous Oxide Mixture	1015	73
Carbon Monoxide	1016	14
Chlorine	1017	27
Chlorodifluoromethane	1018	50
Chloropentafluoroethane	1020	50
Monochloropentafluoroethane	1020	50
Chlorotetrafluoroethane	1021	50
Monochlorotetrafluoroethane	1021	50
Chlorotrifluoromethane	1022	50

Figure 5–6 *Hazardous Materials Injuries* sample index and protocol for ammonia. (*Hazardous Material Injuries: A Handbook for Pre-hospital Care,* Stutz, D.R. and S.J. Janusz, 1988, Bradford Communications Corp.; reproduced with permission.)

PROTOCOL 9

TOXICITY LEVEL 3
PROTECTION LEVEL A

DESCRIPTION (Ammonia)

Ammonia is a colorless gas having an extremely pungent odor. Common household ammonia contains only 5 to 10% ammonia. The primary use for ammonia is in fertilizers.

HEALTH HAZARD

Ammonia is toxic by all routes of exposure. It is a powerful irritant, and contact may result in tissue destruction. Unlike most alkaline materials, ammonia produces systemic effects. Severity of effects is dependent on concentration and duration of exposure.

PROTECTION

These products require full protection and should be EPA Level A. The rescuer should wear chemical resistant encapsulated clothing and self-contained breathing apparatus. Patient care personnel should wear chemical resistant impervious clothing, gloves, shoe covers and self-contained breathing apparatus when caring for field decontaminated victims. As further decontamination occurs, step down to an appropriate respirator. See manufacturer's materials safety data sheets for appropriate materials.

SYMPTOMS

--Deep, corrosive, painful burns with irritation and swelling.
--Eye irritation may be severe.
--Blindness may be temporary or permanent.
--Laryngitis, shortness of breath, chest pain.
--Abdominal pain, nausea, vomiting.
--Shock, pulmonary edema.
--Lightheadedness may precede coma.

Figure 5–6 (*continued*)

PROTOCOL 9

BASIC LIFE SUPPORT
--Remove victim from contaminated atmosphere.
--Remove and isolate contaminated clothing.
--Thoroughly flush exposed eyes with water for 15-30 minutes.
--Decontaminate skin by immediately washing with soapy water.
--Administer oxygen, 6-10 L.
--Administer 1-2 glasses of water or milk to victim following
   ingestion exposure.
--Monitor victim for shock. Treat as necessary.

ADVANCED LIFE SUPPORT
--Initiate IV, Ringer's Lactate (or normal saline), KVO.
--Observe for pulmonary edema. See Appendix B for pulmonary
   edema protocol.

DECONTAMINATION
All clothing should be removed and contained for disposal or
decontamination. Wash the patient with copious amounts of water.
Use of a detergent (such as Tide) is appropriate. Sufficient water
and soap should be used to insure appropriate dilution of the
product. Other solutions may be used as indicated in Appendix G.

PRECAUTIONS
--Administration of an analgesic (for pain) may be necessary.
--DO NOT attempt to neutralize with acids.

Figure 5–6 (*continued*)

Emergency Handling of Hazardous Materials in Surface Transportation. Washington, D.C.: Association of American Railroads, 1981.

This guidebook contains an alphabetic list of the hazardous chemicals most commonly transported by railroad in the United States. It contains a simple summary of fire and reactivity risks. It is useful for establishing initial action plans. It does not provide useful technical or health care information.

ELECTRONIC DATA BASES

In an era of portable computers and cellular telephones, it is possible for emergency responders to access electronic data bases while at the site of hazardous materials emergencies. A growing number of data base sources provide information of potential value to rescue personnel. In general, these data sources provide comprehensive information on the following:

- Physical and chemical properties
- Flammability and reactivity risks
- Choice and use of personal protective equipment
- Health exposure limits
- Hazardous materials regulatory information

Some provide extensive lists of symptoms and health risks; however, few contain comprehensive health care information beyond first-aid techniques.

National Library of Medicine (NLM).   Bethesda, Md.

The NLM offers an extensive assortment of electronic data bases, the majority containing literature references to guide researchers doing library research, although some contain excerpts from published books and scientific journals. MEDLINE and TOXLINE provide literature references. TOXNET, CHEMLINE, and TOXLIT contain excerpts from published books and scientific journals, and also access to data contained in other data bases such as the Chemical Hazards Response Information System (CHRIS), the Registry of Toxic Effects of Chemical Substances, and the Hazardous Substances Databank. In general, the NLM data bases are well maintained and frequently updated, but difficult to use without fairly extensive training.

Hazardline.   Occupational Health Services, Secaucus, N.J.

Hazardline is a commercial data base offering extensive information on more than seventy thousand chemicals. The data base is easy to use and provides useful summaries of the following:

- Physical and chemical properties
- Flammability and reactivity risks

- Choice and use of personal protective equipment
- Advice for containing spills and extinguishing fires
- Health exposure limits
- Simple summaries of health effects
- Lists of symptoms and first-aid responses

The medical treatment information is mostly summarized from a single, standard textbook on poisoning.

Computer-Aided Management of Emergency Operations (CAMEO). *National Oceanographic and Atmospheric Agency, Seattle, Wash.*

CAMEO was designed to provide a complete package of emergency planning and response skills for hazardous materials emergency responders. The data base includes a compilation of first-aid and response information drawn from documents previously published by various governmental agencies. It also provides tools for mapping community hazards, calculating dispersion plumes for planning purposes, and managing right-to-know information required under the SARA. Health care management information contained in CAMEO is primarily simple first-aid techniques.

Chemical Information Systems, Inc. (CIS), *Baltimore, Md.*

CIS provides access to more than thirty different electronic data bases containing scientific, toxicologic, and regulatory information including CHRIS. The scope of available information is great; however, health care management information contains primarily first-aid techniques and directions.

TOMES. *Micromedex, Inc., Denver, Colo.*

TOMES is a series of data bases made available on CD-ROM. It includes first-responder protocols, medical treatment information, hazardous materials management information, and access to four other hazardous materials data bases published by various federal agencies. TOMES has been developed from a toxicology data base used in many poison control centers. It requires a CD-ROM disk drive in addition to a personal computer.

Hazardous Materials Response Database. *Bradford Communications, Beltsville, Md.*

This data base is a companion to *Hazardous Materials Injuries* by Stutz and Janusz described earlier. It contains basic and advanced prehospital EMS protocols for more than three thousand chemicals. It is provided on diskettes in versions for either PC–compatible or Macintosh computers.

TELEPHONE INFORMATION SERVICES

Several organizations provide 24-hour telephone access to technical information about hazardous materials. In most cases, they can be contacted by means of toll-free telephone lines. Emergency responders should maintain up-to-date lists of appropriate telephone numbers as a piece of their basic response equipment.

CHEMTREC. *800-424-9300.*

CHEMTREC is a private service operated by the Chemical Manufacturers Association to provide information on emergency response for chemicals involved in transportation accidents. It also assists emergency responders by providing access to industrial experts, provides nonemergency information on chemicals, and can provide hard copies of information materials.

CANUTEC. *613-966-6666.*

CANUTEC is the Canadian equivalent to CHEMTREC and is operated as a branch of Transport Canada, an agency of the Canadian federal government.

National Response Center (NRC). *800-424-8802.*

Under U.S. federal laws, the NRC must be notified whenever a serious accident involving hazardous materials has occurred. In addition, NRC provides 24-hour assistance to emergency responders in identifying materials and planning emergency responses to accidents.

Agency for Toxic Substances and Disease Registry (ATSDR). *404-488-4100.*

The ATSDR provides 24-hour assistance to physicians and emergency responders who require toxicologic information or guidance for responding to victims of acute hazardous materials exposures. The agency's staff provides a wide range of assistance including treatment protocols, laboratory support, and consultations on chemical activity and toxicology, evacuation planning, public health threat assessment, and decontamination.

Association of American Railroads (AAR). *202-639-2222.*

The AAR provides 24-hour assistance for responding to chemical accidents involving railroad transportation. This organization was previously known as the Bureau of Explosives.

Centers for Disease Control (CDC). *404-633-5313.*

The CDC provides 24-hour assistance to emergency responders who must deal with transportation accidents and damaged packages containing biologic and etiologic hazards such as specimens of bacteria and viruses.

National Pesticide Telecommunications Network (NPTN).   800-858-7378.

The NPTN provides 24-hour assistance to physicians and emergency responders dealing with pesticide exposures and accidents. Information available includes toxicologic data, management and treatment strategies, and procedures for-cleanup after spills and leaks.

Nuclear Regulatory Commission (NRC).   301-951-0550.

The NRC provides 24-hour assistance to emergency responders dealing with accidents involving radioactive materials. This agency can assist in the response to leaks, transportation accidents, and loss or theft of radioactive substances. The agency's staff will also help physicians and EMS personnel to contact appropriate health physicists and other specialists needed for the treatment of radiation victims.

Poison Control Centers (PCC).

About thirty-five regional PCCs are in the United States, each with its own telephone number. To find the telephone number for the nearest PCC, check the local telephone directory or call directory assistance. The PCCs provide 24-hour assistance to physicians and emergency responders dealing with poisonings and acute hazardous materials accidents. Information available includes recommendations for immediate first aid and treatment protocols for exposure victims.

RIGHT-TO-KNOW FORMS

Federal laws and regulations require many companies to provide information about the hazardous materials that they use to their workers and others in the communities around their plants and work sites. The most important of these regulations are included in OSHA's Hazard Communication Standard (HCS) and the SARA. Because emergency responders can expect to receive information on hazardous materials in the form required to achieve compliance with those laws and regulations, responders should become familiar with them.

Hazards Communication Standard

The HCS is an example of a worker right-to-know law. It requires that all employers provide information to workers about the various hazardous chemicals to which they are actually or potentially exposed. The information to be provided is contained in an MSDS, which was described earlier in chapter 4. These information sheets contain summaries of the chemical and physical properties of chemicals, flammability and reactivity data, a brief overview of their health effects, health exposure limits, and instruction for first aid of exposure victims. A sample MSDS is presented as Figure 4–7. Refer to Figure 5–7 for a photograph

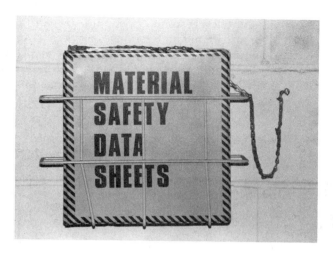

Figure 5–7 This three-ring binder contains material safety data sheets (MSDS) addressing the hazards located in this industrial facility. MSDS forms should be easily accessible to all workers and will be located throughout the plant and with key personnel.

of a three-ring binder containing MSDS forms. This binder has been installed on the wall of a loading dock where hazardous materials are handled.

Superfund Amendments and Reauthorization Act

SARA Title III is an example of a community right-to-know law. It requires that most users of hazardous chemicals provide information about the hazardous materials present in those communities to local emergency planning committees. As a result, emergency responders can now know in advance about the hazardous chemicals to be found at most work sites in their communities.

Moreover, if a significant leak or spill of any of nearly a thousand hazardous chemicals occurs, then SARA requires that an emergency notification be immediately filed to identify that substance, summarize its health effects, and provide advice on the management and treatment strategies for exposure victims. Initially, most emergency notifications will be filed orally. The law requires that written follow-up reports also be submitted. Community emergency responders should be certain to establish a mechanism to receive these filings so that the information is promptly transmitted to personnel at the emergency.

SUMMARY

Once emergency responders recognize and identify hazardous materials at an incident, they must be concerned with collecting enough information to understand the dangers they pose and the specific methods necessary to contain them. EMS responders have the additional task of researching clinical effects and management protocols.

Information sources that are available include books and other printed materials, electronic data bases, emergency information services available by telephone and right-to-know forms. Emergency responders should develop a library of resources with which they are familiar. Response services should establish methods to assure that adequate research information is available at every hazardous materials incident. EMS personnel should work with medical control physicians and hospitals to develop resource libraries and medical protocols for each EMS system.

REFERENCES

BRONSTEIN, A. C., and P. L. CURRANCE, *Emergency Care for Hazardous Materials Exposure.* St. Louis: The C. V. Mosby Company, 1988.

BUNN, W. B., "Right-to-Know Laws and Evaluation of Toxicologic Data." *Ann. Intern. Med.* 103 (1985) 947-49.

CARLSON, GENE P., ed., *HazMat Response Team Leak and Spill Guide.* Stillwater, Okla: Fire Protection Publications, 1984.

Emergency Handling of Hazardous Materials in Surface Transportation. Washington, D.C.: Association of American Railroads, 1981.

1987 Emergency Response Guidebook. Washington, D.C.: U.S. Department of Transportation, 1987.

"Extremely Hazardous Substances List and Threshold Planning Quantities: Emergency Planning and Release Notification Requirements: Final Rule." *Federal Register,* 52 (April 22, 1987), 13378–410.

"Hazard Communication: Final Rule." *Federal Register,* 48 (November 25, 1983), 53280–347.

LEFÈVRE, M. J., *First Aid Manual for Chemical Accidents.* New York: Van Nostrand Reinhold Co., 1980.

Medical First Aid Guide for Use in Accidents Involving Dangerous Goods. Geneva: International Maritime Organization, 1985.

MEYER, E., *Chemistry of Hazardous Materials.* Englewood Cliffs, N.J.: Brady Books, 1989.

MORGAN, D. P.: *Recognition and Management of Pesticide Poisonings.* Washington, D.C.: U.S. Environmental Protection Agency, 1982.

NIOSH Pocket Guide to Chemical Hazards. Washington, D.C.: U.S. Department of Health and Human Services, 1985.

NOLL, G. G ., M. S. HILDEBRAND, and J. G. YVORRA, *Hazardous Materials: Managing the Incident.* Stillwater, Okla.: Fire Protection Publications, 1988.

PROCTOR, N. H., J. P. HUGHES, and M. L. FISCHMAN, *Chemical Hazards of the Workplace.* Philadelphia: J.B. Lippincott Company, 1988.

SAX, N. I., and R. J. LEWIS, *Dangerous Properties of Industrial Materials.* New York: Van Nostrand Reinhold Co., 1989.

STUTZ, D. R., and S. J. JANUSZ, *Hazardous Materials Injuries: A Handbook for Pre-Hospital Care.* Beltsville, Md.: Bradford Communications, 1988.

DETECTION INSTRUMENTATION

CHAPTER 6

GOAL: On completion of this chapter the student will understand the role of detection instruments in the initial response to a hazardous materials incident.

OBJECTIVES:

Specifically, the student will be able to

- Describe the role of combustible gas indicators
- Name the two commonest reference gases
- Name one limitation of a combustible gas indicator
- Describe the role of oxygen meters
- Describe the role of colorimetric tubes
- Describe the role of radiation meters
- Describe the role of pH detectors
- Describe the role of dosimeters
- Discuss the limitations of detection instruments

OVERVIEW

It is often possible to recognize and identify the hazardous materials that are present at an accident site. Some of the clues that indicate their presence, and the labels and warning placards that identify them were described earlier (see chapter 4). Unfortunately, the information that can be obtained from clues and labels is insufficient to characterize the emergency fully in most cases. It is often valuable for responders to know the concentrations of chemicals present in the atmosphere at an accident. It is also important for them to determine how widely a spilled chemical has dispersed.

Emergency responders need to use detection instruments to measure the levels of contamination at a hazardous materials accident, to evaluate the extent of chemical dispersion, and to identify otherwise unknown toxic chemicals. These devices can provide an assortment of useful information. In this chapter the role of such instruments will be discussed in the initial response to a hazardous material incident. Then six types of metering devices will be described. Finally, some of the cautions that should be observed when using these instruments will be reviewed.

ROLE OF DETECTION INSTRUMENTS

A major role of detectors is to help identify the actual hazards involved at an accident. The importance of identifying the hazardous materials at an accident site has been described in several previous chapters. Responders must know when they are confronted by hazards and dangers so that appropriate protective actions can be taken. EMS and other medical personnel should know which hazards have affected victims so that the most appropriate emergency health care can be provided.

It is also important that responders know the air concentrations of toxic gases and vapors at an incident to determine the need for personal protective equipment and the types of equipment that are necessary. These concerns are discussed in chapter 7. For example, air purification respirators are only effective for specific chemicals and over narrowly defined concentration ranges. Without knowing the precise chemical identity and its concentration level, rescuers should not wear respirators and must use self-contained breathing apparatus (SCBA). Likewise, the choice of protective clothing also depends on the air concentration of the toxic chemicals. If responders must enter a potentially lethal environment, such as one with chemical concentrations in excess of the IDLH level, they must wear chemical protective clothing. Accordingly, a second role of detection instruments is to help determine which protective equipment should be used and when it can be removed.

Another role for detection instruments is the identification of other types of hazardous conditions, such as explosion and fire risks or oxygen deficiency. Because more than 65 percent of hazardous materials are flammable and explosive, responders must frequently face the possibility of fire or explosion. By measuring the air concentrations of combustible gases, it is possible to determine whether those gases are present in their flammable (explosive) ranges (see chapter 3). If a gas is approaching that range, then a fire or explosion threat is present, and responders must take extensive precautions.

Oxygen deficiency can occur because of chemical reactions or fires that use up the available oxygen. It can also result from the leak of a heavier-than-air gas, which displaces the oxygen and air from a closed space or room. Responders who enter an oxygen-deficient environment without an independent air supply can quickly suffer asphyxia and death.

Still other roles for detection instruments include evaluation of radiation accidents and measurement of the pH at accidents involving acids and alkali. Radiation detectors and survey meters are necessary to determine the presence of radiation at an accident involving radioactive materials. Measurements of pH can help identify the nature of a spilled corrosive liquid. In monitoring the adequacy of decontamination and washing contaminated eyes and skin, pH measurements are also useful (see chapters 16 and 17).

COMBUSTIBLE GAS INDICATORS

Combustible gas indicators, or explosimeters, measure the air concentration of a flammable gas or vapor for which the indicator has been specifically calibrated. Refer to Figure 6–1 for examples of two of the commonest types of combustible gas indicators. Most indicators are calibrated for either hexane or methane, which are then known as the *reference gas.* To operate the indicator, a sample of air to be tested is drawn into a combustion chamber within the meter by means of a pump or aspirator. As the air is drawn in, it passes over a heated platinum filament wire, which combusts the airborne gas. The burning gas gives off heat, which the indicator measures and converts into an estimate of the air concentration of that combustible substance.

By convention, these instruments yield results that are stated in terms of the LEL (see chapter 3) of the calibrated gas. For example, such an instrument may indicate that the air concentration of methane is 20, 50, or 100 percent of methane's LEL. As the percentage of the LEL increases, so does the danger of an explosion. See Figure 6–2 for an example of this concept.

Combustible gas indicators are most accurate when used to detect the specific reference gas for which the indicator has been calibrated. Determinations of the concentrations of other gases require conversion tables or reference curves, and results are usually less accurate. These indicators do not function properly in oxygen-deficient or oxygen-enriched atmospheres. In either situation, abnormal oxygen concentrations will cause the reference gas to combust at either a lower or higher temperature than expected; the detection instrument will, therefore, yield inaccurate results.

OXYGEN METERS

Oxygen meters measure the proportion of oxygen in the surrounding atmosphere. At sea level, oxygen normally makes up about 21 percent of the air. At higher altitudes the air contains less oxygen. The concentration of oxygen in the

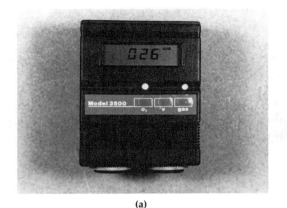

(a)

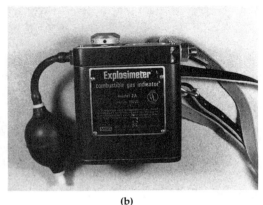

(b)

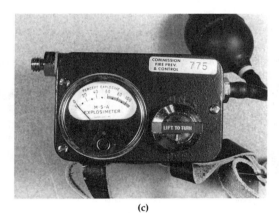

(c)

Figure 6–1 Two of the more common types of combustible gas indicators. (a) Biosystems 3500 Meter (Biosystems, Rockfall, CT) has a digital readout. (b) MSA Explosimeter (Mine Safety Appliances Co., Pittsburgh, Pa.), top view, with a scaled dial 0–100% of the lower explosive limit. (c) MSA Explosimeter, side view.

air also varies slightly with the barometric pressure. An oxygen proportion in air of less than 19.5 percent will pose a life- and health-threatening situation to rescuers or victims who are not equipped with an independent air supply. As oxygen deficiency worsens, asphyxia and death can occur quickly.

Oxygen meters operate by drawing air through a membrane and allowing the oxygen to react with a sensitive electrolyte solution, which results in the generation of an electrical charge. Such meters are often coupled with combustible gas indicators and are known as combination meters. These meters should be calibrated before each use so as to compensate for changing altitude and barometric pressure. False readings can result from exposure of the meter to environments containing halogen gases such as chlorine or CO_2.

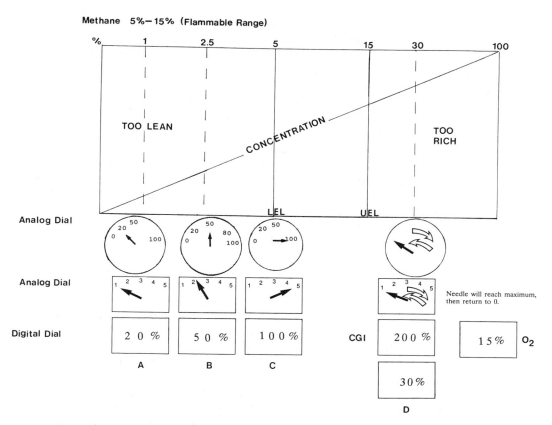

Figure 6–2 An illustration of the three most common dials on a CGI (combustible gas indicator). Analog scales can be 0–100% of the lower explosive limit (LEL) or a direct reading of methane in air (5% = LEL). The digital dial gives a numeric reading of the percentage approaching the LEL. Point A shows readings that correlate to 20% of the LEL. Ignition cannot occur because the concentration is too lean. Point B shows readings that are 50% of the LEL; ignition cannot occur, however, the atmosphere is approaching serious and dangerous levels. Point C's meter indicates that the LEL has been reached; an explosion or ignition can occur. Point D's meter shows what will occur when the concentration is too rich. The meter's reading will rise to a maximum reading and then decrease to either 0 or the chemical's concentration in air (example: 30% methane in air). A corresponding decrease in oxygen will also register if the meter has an oxygen reading capability.

COLORIMETRIC TUBES

Colorimetric tubes are used to determine the presence and approximate concentration of many chemicals that might be present in the atmosphere to be tested. For each suspected chemical, a unique and specific colorimetric tube exists.

These tubes are sealed glass vials containing small amounts of reactive chemicals. After breaking open the tube ends, a measured amount of air is drawn through the tube by means of a bellows or pump. If the suspected chemical is present in the air, it reacts with the tube's contents to cause a measurable color change. Figure 6-3 illustrates three types of colorimetric tubes.

The amount of color change that results when a known volume of air is drawn through a colorimetric tube determines the approximate air concentration of the chemical. These results are only approximations, however. The amount of color change can be influenced by the temperature of the contaminated place, the age of the tube, and the presence of more than one contaminating chemical.

Colorimetric tubes are manufactured by several companies. Each manufacturer's tubes are used in slightly different ways and can yield somewhat different results. Before using any specific set of tubes, responders should review the instructions that are enclosed in the tube package. This will assure proper use of the tubes, and readings will be as accurate as possible.

RADIATION METERS

Radiation meters are used to detect the presence and measure the quantity of radiation emitted by the decay of radioactive substances. Radioactive decay emits at least three types of radiation: alpha particles, beta particles, and gamma rays. Gamma radiation is a form of electromagnetic energy that is similar to but more powerful than most x-rays and microwaves. Gamma radiation is generally measured by use of Geiger counters. Beta particles are roughly equivalent to high-speed electrons and can be measured using a "thin-window" Geiger counter. Alpha particles are indistinguishable from the nuclei of helium atoms. Geiger counters do not detect alpha particles, for which special metering devices are usually required. A Geiger counter and dosimeter are illustrated in Figure 6-4.

When charged radioactive particles or ionizing radiation pass through the sensing chamber of a radiation meter, they cause atoms of the gas within the chamber to become ionized and unstable. That allows an electrical pulse to flow across the chamber. The radiation meter measures the resulting electrical current and converts it into an estimate of the amount of radiation in the environment.

pH DETECTORS

The pH is a measure of the acidity-alkalinity of a substance. It is based on a scale that runs from 0 (most acidic) to 14 (most alkaline). Solutions with a pH of 7 are neutral and have neither acidic nor alkaline qualities. The normal body pH is about 7.4. Substances that have a low pH (below pH of 2) and those with a high

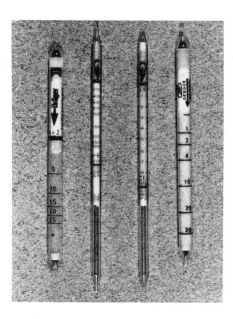

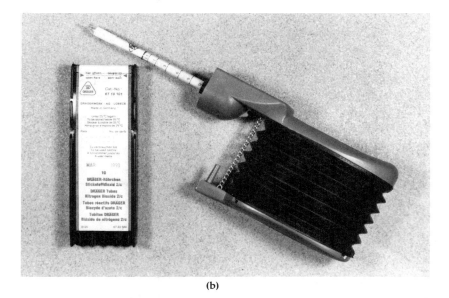

(b)

Figure 6–3 Various types of colorimetric tubes. (a) Different types of tubes from different manufacturers. Outside tubes are Draeger® (National Draeger, Inc., Pittsburgh, Pa.); inside tubes are Gastec® (Sensidyne, Inc., Largo, Fla.), MSA (Mine Safety Appliances Co., Pittsburgh, Pa.), and Sensidyne® (Sensidyne, Inc., Largo, Fla.). (b) A common type of bellows used to draw air through the colorimetric tubes. This example is manufactured by Draeger.

pH (greater than 11.5) are capable of causing severe damage to living tissues. The tissue effects of strong acids and alkali are discussed in chapters 15 and 16.

Simple determinations of pH can be made using litmus paper, pH paper, or laboratory "dip sticks," which undergo color changes that depend on the acidity or alkalinity of the solutions with which they are moistened. More sophisticated and precise determinations can be made using electronic pH meters. The use of a pH dip stick to measure the pH of the eye is shown later in chapter 13 (see Figure 13–3). Dip sticks and pH paper provide a simple means for monitoring the adequacy of decontamination and removal of acids and alkali from the skin and eyes of exposure victims. Some common types of electronic pH meters are shown in Figure 6–5.

SAMPLING DEVICES

The most accurate measurements of environmental contamination and personal exposure are achieved when samples of contaminated air or water are subjected to rigorous laboratory evaluations. The results of such testing are not generally useful for emergency responders who must act within a time frame that rarely permits laboratory studies. The use of dosimeters can occasionally be helpful in determining whether exposure victims need complex medical treatments. Dosimeters are badgelike meters that are worn by workers and others who are at risk of exposure to high levels of radiation or specific toxic chemicals. These devices provide an accurate measure of the total exposure suffered by a person; however, the results may not be immediately available. In the case of delayed

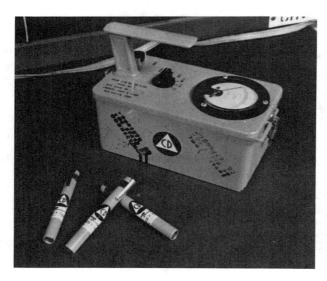

Figure 6–4 Two of the most common types of radiologic monitoring devices: Geiger counter and dosimeter.

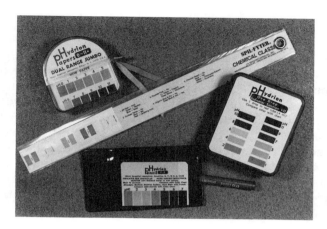

Figure 6–5 Some of the most common types of pH detectors that are available to responders.

acting hazards such as phosgene, knowledge of the total exposure dose can permit physicians to determine whether victims require hospitalization.

CAUTIONS ABOUT DETECTION INSTRUMENTS

The information obtained by using detection instruments is prone to errors and inaccuracies. Combustible gas indicators and colorimetric tubes may provide confusing information for numerous reasons. Cross-reactions can occur between chemicals of similar type. A tube meant for detecting methanol, for example, will show a reactive color change when exposed to ethanol. Errors can result from the use of out-of-date tubes or poorly calibrated gas indicators. Inaccurate combustible gas indicator readings can be due to filament damage that results when an indicator is used in an oxygen-enriched atmosphere. For these and other reasons, the information obtained by using detection instruments should be regarded as no better than approximations. When the results of metering by several different methods are available to responders, they should use the most conservative set as the basis for decisions regarding safety precautions and protective equipment.

All detection instruments have concentration thresholds below which they cannot detect the presence of chemicals. As a result, a negative or ''zero'' result of testing does not necessarily indicate that the tested area is clean. It is possible that such negative results indicate only a low level of contamination. In addition, contamination conditions can change depending on the activity at a site as well as the site's temperature, wind speed, and humidity. Accordingly, testing and monitoring should be repeated regularly during an emergency response to assure that safety precautions and selected protective equipment remain appropriate.

SUMMARY

Detection instruments are important devices for identifying and quantifying the hazards involved at a hazardous materials incident. The information provided can be critical for choosing appropriate protective equipment and avoiding unexpected hazards such as fires, explosions and oxygen-deficient environments.

Useful detection instruments include combustible gas indicators, oxygen meters, colorimetric tubes, radiation meters, pH meters, and sampling devices. Emergency responders should become familiar with the operations of each of these types of detection equipment. It is also important that the limitations of each device be well understood. The careful and proper use of detection instruments can permit responders to protect themselves better from exposure to hazardous materials.

REFERENCES

"Air Sampling Instruments for Evaluation of Atmospheric Contaminants" (American Conference of Governmental Industrial Hygienists, Cincinnati, Ohio, 1989).

CARLSON, GENE P., ed., *HazMat Response Team Leak and Spill Guide.* Stillwater, Okla.: Fire Protection Publications, Oklahoma State University, 1984.

COSTELLO, R. J., *NIOSH Health Hazard Evaluations Determination Report HETA 83-417-1357,* pp. 6–7, Bridge City, Tex.: U.S. Environmental Protection Agency Triangle Chemical Site, 1983.

COSTELLO, R. J., B. FROENBERG, and J. MELIUS, *Health Hazard Evaluation Determination Report,* Rollins Environmental Services, Baton Rouge, La., HE 81-37. Cincinnati, Ohio: National Institute for Occupational Safety and Health, 1981.

COSTELLO, R. J., and J. MELIUS, *Technical Assistance Determination Report, Chemical Control,* Elizabeth, N.J. TA 80-77, pp 20-22, Cincinnati, Ohio: National Institute for Occupational Safety and Health, 1981.

Direct Reading Colorimetric Indicator Tubes Manual. Akron, Ohio: American Industrial Hygiene Association, 1988.

Emergency Control of Hazardous Materials Incidents II. N.Y.: Office of Fire Prevention and Control, State of New York, Department of State, Albany, 1988.

Fundamentals of Industrial Hygiene. Chicago, Ill.: National Safety Council, 1988.

HILL, R. H., and J. E. ARNOLD, "A Personal Air Sampler for Pesticides," *Arch. Envir. Contam. Toxicol., 8 (1979),* 621–28.

Manual of Recommended Practice for Combustible Gas Indicators and Portable, Direct Reading Hydrocarbon Detectors. Akron, Ohio: American Industrial Hygiene Association, 1987.

NIOSH, *Manual of Analytical Methods* (4th ed.), Springfield, Va.: NTIS, National Institute for Occupational Safety and Health, 1984.

Occupational Safety and Health Guidance Manual for Hazardous Waste Site Activities. Washington, D.C.: NIOSH/OSHA/USCG/EPA, U.S. Department of Health and Human Services, 1985.

OSHA, *Industrial Hygiene Technical Manual,* OSHA Instruction CPL 2-2.20A. Washington, D.C., OSHA, 1984.

Standard Operating Safety Guides. Washington, D.C., Environmental Response Branch, Hazardous Response Support Division, Office of Emergency and Remedial Response, U.S. Environmental Protection Agency, 1984.

PERSONAL PROTECTIVE EQUIPMENT

CHAPTER 7

GOAL: On completion of this chapter the student will be able to discuss the role of personal protective equipment in a hazardous materials incident.

OBJECTIVES:

Specifically, the student will be able to

- Name the two types of respiratory protection
- Describe the function of air purification devices
- Discuss the limitations of air purification devices
- Describe the function of air supply devices
- Discuss the criteria for choosing between self-contained breathing apparatus or airline hoses
- Name the four-stage classification of chemical protective clothing (CPC) developed by the EPA
- Describe the characteristics of each level of protection
- Discuss the characteristics of fully encapsulating and nonencapsulating CPC and the advantages and disadvantages of each
- Name the two major classes of materials from which CPC are manufactured and give examples of each
- Discuss the qualities emergency responders should look for when choosing CPC
- Name the three ways in which hazardous materials enter CPC
- Define breakthrough time
- Define permeation rate

OVERVIEW

The emergency response to a hazardous materials incident will sometimes require that response personnel risk exposure to potentially dangerous concentrations of toxic chemicals. To accomplish their tasks, emergency responders may need to enter areas of high contamination deliberately where unprotected exposures would likely prove fatal. To do this, personnel must use specialized clothing and respiratory protection that offers adequate protection from the harmful effects of contaminating chemicals.

Choosing the right protective clothing and equipment to use at a hazardous materials incident is an important aspect of the emergency response plan. In some hazardous materials situations no appropriate protection may be available. For most, however, at least several acceptable alternatives from which to choose will be available. Critical to these choices are the actual hazards to be dealt with, their likely concentrations, and the form in which the hazards will be found.

In this chapter, the types of protective equipment and clothing that are generally available, some criteria for choosing among them, and the advantages and disadvantages of each will be reviewed. Also discussed will be some concepts of protection and the ways by which protection can be measured and quantified. Finally, these general concepts will be related to issues of specific relevance to EMS and other health care personnel.

RESPIRATORY PROTECTION

Inhalation exposure poses the greatest risk to emergency responders at a hazardous materials accident. A danger of direct toxic injury to the lungs and airways exists as well as a danger that inhaled toxins will be absorbed and cause systemic poisoning. Respiratory exposure to high concentrations of some toxins, such as ammonia or hydrogen cyanide, can cause death after only a breath or two. Other hazardous chemicals, such as cadmium, can lead to toxic reactions that evolve slowly following inhalation exposure. Direct toxic effects on the lungs and airways by inhaled chemicals are described later in chapter 15, and the systemic effects of inhaled toxins are described in chapter 18.

Protection of the respiratory system can be accomplished by removing hazardous substances from the inhaled air or by providing uncontaminated air to the rescue personnel who must function in contaminated areas. Both approaches, air purification and air supply, have advantages and disadvantages that are described subsequently.

Air Purification Devices

Air purification devices consist of filters or respirators that remove foreign materials and chemicals from the inhaled air. Their actual shape and design may

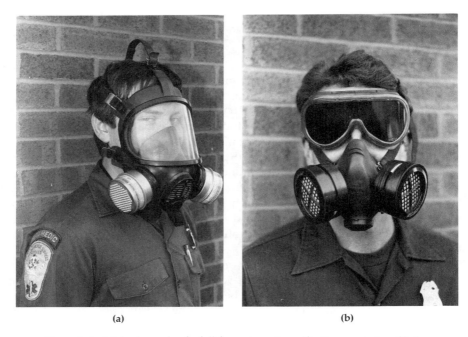

(a)   (b)

Figure 7–1 (a) An example of a full-face–piece air purification respirator. (b) An example of a half-face–piece air purification respirator with goggles.

vary, but all work on a simple principle that requires the wearer to draw air across the filtration system with each breath. Two types of air purification respirators are shown in Figure 7–1. They are generally portable and simple to use. Unfortunately, their value is severely limited because of the following concerns:

- Respirator filters are generally designed to be used in the presence of a specific chemical. They are often ineffective if used for protection against other chemicals. For this reason, air purification devices should not be used when contamination is due to unidentified toxins or mixed toxins.

- Respirator filters are generally effective over only a limited range of chemical concentrations. Use of a respirator may not be safe unless the actual chemical air concentrations have been measured and found to be within the respirator's effective range.

- Respirator filters are usually calibrated for use at room temperature, and they may not function adequately when used at elevated temperatures and at fire scenes.

- Respirator filters have limited and uncertain durations of effectiveness that depend on the ways in which they have been stored.

For these and other technical reasons, filter respirators should not be used routinely by first responders at hazardous materials incidents. They should only be used following identification of the specific hazards involved and measurement of their atmospheric concentrations have determined that use of a filter respirator is safe.

Air Supply Devices

Air supply devices protect response personnel against the dangers of both inhaled toxins and oxygen deficiency. Lack of oxygen can occur during fires, which use up available oxygen, and after closed-space leaks of heavier-than-air gases that displace oxygen. Air supply devices provide compressed air, at pressures that are greater than atmospheric pressure, to a face mask that is worn by the rescuer. Air can be supplied by compressed air tanks (SCBAs), or airline hoses. A rescuer in chemical protective clothing and equipped with SCBA is shown in Figure 7–2.

Positive pressure air supply devices provide greater protection than filter respirators and should be used by first responders and rescue personnel at incidents involving unidentified hazards, mixed hazards, and high-concentration hazards. The decision to use SCBA or airline hoses should be based on practical considerations such as the following:

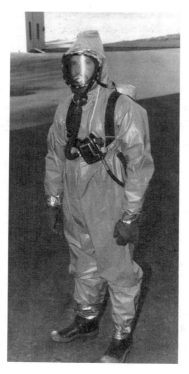

Figure 7–2 A typical air supply respirator commonly referred to as a *self-contained breathing apparatus*. In this example, the rescuer is also wearing chemical protective clothing.

- Airline hoses restrict the mobility of rescuers.
- Airline hoses require that rescuers retrace their entry path as they exit so that the hose can be brought out of the contaminated area.
- Airline hoses can be damaged, thus endangering the rescuer who is using it.
- As the length of airline hose increases, the air pressure that reaches the face mask can fall dangerously. The maximum airline hose length approved by the NIOSH is 300 feet.
- SCBA provides limited volumes of air and, therefore, rescuers usually have only a limited air supply for continuous working in the contaminated area. By contrast, airline hoses can provide unlimited amounts of air.

Emergency response personnel should use respiratory protective equipment with which they are familiar. Regular practice and drills with airway equipment is essential to assure that equipment and personnel function properly together. During an actual emergency is the wrong time to learn how to operate a new piece of equipment. Backup air packs or airline hoses should always be available before entry is made by rescuers into an oxygen-deficient or IDLH environment. A backup team of rescuers with equal or greater protection must also be prepared to enter the contaminated area in the event that failure of air supply equipment threatens the loss of one of the original entry team.

CHEMICAL PROTECTIVE CLOTHING

CPC encompasses a wide assortment of equipment that ranges from standard work uniforms to highly specialized clothing ensembles capable of resisting attack by many chemicals as well as heat and fire. Emergency responders must choose from a broad selection of alternative styles and types of CPC constructed of differing materials and fabrics. Ultimately, the choice of CPC to use at a specific incident is dictated by the chemical hazards to be confronted, their likely concentrations, and the probability that rescuers will suffer skin contamination.

Before responders begin to choose or use CPC, however, they should understand the levels of protection that different types of equipment can offer, the advantages and disadvantages of various CPC fabrics and designs, and the limitations and risks of each. These concerns will be discussed in the following sections.

LEVELS OF PROTECTION

A four-stage classification of chemical protective clothing, which is based on the levels of protection provided by types of equipment, has been developed by the EPA. This classification system does not describe specific equipment. Instead, it defines categories, or Levels, according to the situational needs of hazardous materials workers and the goals of the equipment to be used. By this system, the highest level of protection is called Level A, and the lowest is Level D. The EPA terminology has become widely accepted and types of CPC are often referred to according to corresponding EPA Levels from A to D.

Level A

Level A protection is required for entry into areas of high contamination that pose risks of inhalation, skin, mucous membrane, and eye exposure. This level of protection is required for toxic environments that exceed the IDLH level and for prolonged work at contamination levels greater than the STEL. To achieve Level A protection, CPC must include at least the following:

- Positive-pressure SCBA
- Fully encapsulating chemical-resistant suit
- Double layer of chemical-resistant gloves
- Chemical-resistant boots
- Airtight seals between the suit, and the gloves and boots

See Figure 7–3 for a photograph of a Level A suit.

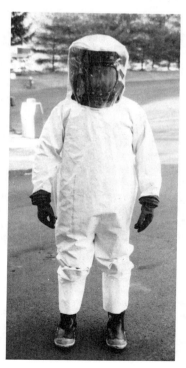

Figure 7–3 A totally encapsulating Level A suit. The glove ring assembly and integral bootie make a unit capable of holding test pressures in accordance with ASTM FS93.

Level B

Level B equipment provides respiratory protection comparable to Level A, but lesser protection against skin, mucous membrane, and eye exposures. Level B CPC suits are chemical resistant and offer protection against splash exposures. They are not fully encapsulating, however, and may allow vapors and dusts to enter at the neck, wrists, and closures. Level B protection is the minimum level that should be used for entry into a hazardous material site that has not been fully tested and monitored. Refer to Figure 7–4 for examples of Level B protective clothing.

To achieve Level B protection, CPC must include at least the following:

- Positive-pressure SCBA
- Chemical-resistant, long-sleeved suit
- Double layer of chemical-resistant gloves
- Chemical resistant boots

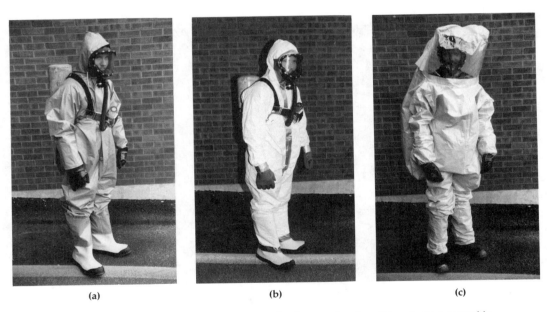

(a)   (b)   (c)

Figure 7–4 Level B protection. (a) An example of a one-piece Level B protection ensemble with self-contained breathing apparatus. Taping of wrists, ankles, and face piece add protection but should not be substituted for Level A protection. (b) Another form of Level B protection is the single use (disposable) fully encapsulated protective suit. Although this suit resembles a Level A ensemble, it provides only Level B protection and should not be substituted for Level A protection. (c) Level B single-use (disposable) suit with self-contained breathing apparatus.

Level C

Level C equipment is appropriate for use when the hazardous materials have been identified, their concentrations in air are known to fall within the effective range of air purification filters, and little likelihood exists of exposure of the skin, mucous membranes, or eyes. Examples of Level C protective clothing are illustrated in Figure 7–5.

To achieve Level C protection, CPC must include at least the following:

- Full-face, air purification device (respirator)
- Chemical-resistant suit
- Chemical-resistant outer gloves
- Chemical-resistant boots

Level D

Level D equipment is essentially common work clothes that do not provide specific respiratory or skin protection. This level of CPC should not be worn alone

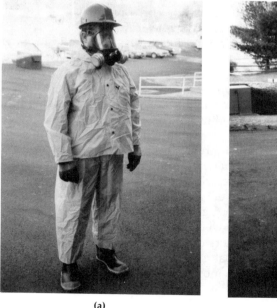
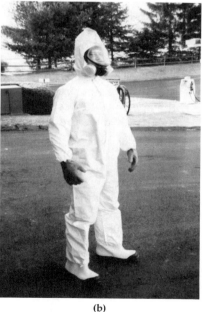

(a)   (b)

Figure 7–5 Two forms of Level C protection. (a) Multiuse two-piece garment. (b) One-piece, single-use TYVEK® (The Du Pont Company, Wilmington, DE)-polyethylene protective clothing with respirator.

in any environment that poses a hazardous materials risk as a result of respiratory, skin, mucous membrane, or eye exposure.

TYPES OF CHEMICAL PROTECTIVE CLOTHING

Chemical protective clothing ensembles are often described as being either fully encapsulating or nonencapsulating. Each type has advantages and disadvantages. Fully encapsulating suits, for example, provide greater amounts of protection but restrict the movements and activities of the wearer. Emergency responders should understand the relative merits of both types of CPC.

Fully Encapsulating Chemical Protective Clothing

Fully encapsulating chemical protective clothing encloses the wearer in a one-piece, airtight structure. Their use is indicated for entry into environments that contain extremely hazardous substances that threaten skin exposure and environments containing unidentified hazardous substances. Protection is offered against chemicals in the form of gases, vapors, mists, or particulate matter in the air. These suits are designed to prevent skin contact that can lead to massive tissue destruction (as can be caused by corrosives such as acids and alkali) or absorption resulting in systemic toxicity (as can result from hydrogen cyanide).

All parts of the suit (including the gloves, boots, and face mask) are integrated into a single structure. In some, the gloves and boots are detachable, whereas in others they are not. Suit closures, usually zippers with overseals, are designed to prevent entry of contaminated air into the suit. Depending on the specific suit design, SCBA may be worn inside or outside of the suit, and a means for attaching an airline hose to the suit may exist.

The ultimate protection provided by these suits depends on the material from which they are made. Different materials provide protection against different chemicals. The various materials used in the manufacture of CPC and the basis for their selection are described in a later section of this chapter.

The advantage of a fully encapsulating suit is the high degree of protection that it provides. The disadvantages include decreased mobility and maneuverability caused by the suits as well as decreased visibility from inside the suits. Responders wearing these suits are generally unable to communicate verbally to others; therefore, they must carry communication devices such as small radios within the suits. Because most suits have no means of ventilation, a danger of heat accumulation exists, causing responders to suffer heat stress and heat stroke. Cooling devices can minimize the dangers of heat accumulation. These suits, however, should be worn by only well-conditioned persons who are well hydrated at the time that they begin using the CPC.

Nonencapsulating CPC

Nonencapsulating CPC is designed to provide protection against respiratory exposures and chemical splash exposures. This type of CPC does not protect against skin exposure to vapors, gases, and airborne dusts. These suits are designed for use in environments that do not contain high air concentrations of extremely hazardous substances. They can also be used when skin, mucous membrane, and eye exposures are unlikely and will not lead to local or systemic toxicity.

Nonencapsulating CPC outfits may consist of a two-piece "splash suit" or a one-piece coverall. The gloves, boots, and face mask are not integrated into the suit; they do not provide protection against the entry of gases, vapors, and dust at the wrists, ankles, and neck of the outfit. Some responders use tape to seal the wrist, ankle, and zipper closures of these CPC more securely. Such use of tape cannot create a fully encapsulating suit equivalent to a Level A ensemble.

Among the advantages of nonencapsulating suits is that they allow mobility and freedom of movement, are relatively easy to put on and take off, and are generally much less expensive than fully encapsulating suits. Their disadvantage is the limited protection that they offer to wearers.

PROTECTIVE MATERIALS AND FABRICS

Chemical protective clothing can be manufactured from several different materials and fabrics that each have different qualities and protective values. These materials are often divided into two major classes: elastomers and nonelastomers. Elastomers are polymer fabrics such as polyvinyl alcohol, Viton® (The Du Pont Company, Wilmington, DE.), butyl rubber neoprene, and nitrile rubber. These are often resistant materials that are employed in reusable CPC. Nonelastomers are generally nonwoven fabrics such as Tyvek® (The Du Pont Company, Wilmington, DE.) and Chemrel® (Chemron, Inc., Buffalo Grove, IL.) that are often used for disposable CPC.

No one material or fabric can provide universal chemical protection. Accordingly, responders must choose CPC on the basis of the specific range of chemical resistance provided by the suit material and other related qualities. In selecting a CPC material or fabric, the following considerations should be of importance to emergency responders:

- Chemical resistance
- Durability
- Flexibility
- Service life

- Ease of decontamination
- Temperature resistance
- Cost

Chemical Resistance

Chemical resistance refers to the ability of a suit fabric or material to prevent harmful chemicals from entering the suit. When a suit material has high resistance to the entry of a specific chemical, it is said to have excellent *chemical compatibility*. Conversely, a material that does not prevent entry by a chemical is said to have poor chemical compatibility. The selection of suit materials for use with specific chemicals is often based on published chemical compatibility charts and recommendations. A section from the *Permeation Guide for Du Pont Protective Apparel Fabrics* is shown in Figure 7–6.

Issues of chemical resistance and chemical compatibility are of primary importance to proper CPC selection. These issues, which should be understood by any responder who is likely to use CPC during a hazardous materials incident, will be discussed in detail later in this chapter.

Durability

The ability of a CPC to resist tearing and punctures is of particular importance. When a suit is torn or punctured, it can no longer protect the wearer. Elastomers tend to be thicker and more durable than nonelastomers; however, recent technical advances have resulted in the development of synthetic nonelastomers with great durability such as Barricade® (The Du Pont Company, Wilmington, DE.) and Responder® (Lifeguard, Inc., Guntersville, AL.).

Flexibility

The flexibility and elasticity of a material determines the ease with which a responder can work while wearing a suit. Stiff materials decrease mobility and dexterity. This consideration is important when choosing gloves. For example, natural rubber is flexible and used for gloves that permit great dexterity. By contrast, polyvinyl alcohol is resistant to many chemicals that penetrate rubber. When used in manufacturing, the product is clumsy, stiff, and hard to use.

Service Life

Some CPC materials suffer aging even when not used. As a result, suits can lose their chemical resistance. Suits with longer shelf life are generally more expensive but may be a better choice for services that anticipate only rare use of CPC equipment. Before CPC are purchased, equipment manufacturers should be consulted regarding shelf life by services anticipating only infrequent use.

Figure 7-6 *Permeation Guide for Du Pont Apparel Fabrics.* The most effective protective clothing combines long breakthrough times with low permeation rates. (Reproduced with permission from The Du Pont Company, Wilmington, DE).

Chemical permeation data

Chemical challenge	TYVEK® QC Coated with 1.25 mil Polyethylene — Breakthrough Time (min.)	Permeation Rate (mg/m²/sec.)	TYVEK® SARANEX®-23P Single Ply — Breakthrough Time (min.)	Permeation Rate (mg/m²/sec.)	TYVEK® SARANEX®-23P Two Ply — Breakthrough Time (min.)	Permeation Rate (mg/m²/sec.)	BARRICADE® — Breakthrough Time (min.)	Permeation Rate (mg/m²/sec.)
N,N-Dimethylformamide, 99+%	30	.1834	120	3.0	>480	nd	203	0.3306
*Dimethylhydrazine, 98%	nt	nt	12	~1	nt	nt	>480	nd
*Epichlorohydrin, 99%	nt	nt	57	8.7	nt	nt	nt	nt
2-Ethoxyethanol, 99%	nt	nt	>480	nd	nt	nt	>480	nd
Ethoxyethyl acetate, 98%	nt	nt	39	0.3	nt	nt	nt	nt
Ethyl acetate, 99%	<1	2.1171	36	1.1	130	0.9	>480	nd
Ethylbenzene, 99+%	nt	nt	nt	nt	nt	nt	nt	nt
Ethyl Cellosolve® 99%	nt	nt	>480	nd	nt	nt	>480	nd
Ethylenediamine, 99%	15	1.7	>480	nd	nt	nt	nt	nt
Ethylene dichloride, 99+%	nt	nt	nt	nt	nt	nt	>480	nd
Ethylene glycol, 99+%	>480	nd	>480	nd	nt	nt	nt	nt
Ethylene oxide gas, 98-100%	0.3	3	6	1.4	55	1.32	>480	nd
Fluorosulfonic acid	10	nm	360	nm	nt	nt	nt	nt
Formaldehyde, 37-40%	>480	nd	>480	nd	nt	nt	nt	nt
Formic acid, 95-97%	4	0.055	>480	nd	nt	nt	>480	nd
Freon 113, 98%	nt	nt	nt	nt	nt	nt	>480	nd
Gasoline, leaded	nt	nt	nt	nt	nt	nt	nt	nt
Hexamethylene diisocyanate, 98%	nt	nt	>480	nd	nt	nt	>480	nd
*n-Hexane, 99%	<1	nm	2	0.005	nt	nt	>311	<0.0018
*Hydrazine, 98%	nt	nt	>480	nd	nt	nt	>480	nd
Hydrochloric acid, 37%	35	nm	>480	nd	nt	nt	>480	nd
Hydrochloric acid, 50%	>30	<0.0005	>480	<0.000077	nt	nt	nt	nt
Hydrofluoric acid anhydrous, 10°C	13	0.001	>30	<0.0008	nt	nt	nt	nt
Hydrofluoric acid anhydrous, 25°C	7	1	20	0.005	nt	nt	nt	nt
Iodine solid, 100%	>420	8	>480	0.5	nt	nt	nt	nt
Jet A fuel	nt	nt	458	18.2	nt	nt	>480	nd
Mercury, 99+%	1	.3667	>210	<.000077	nt	nt	106	0.2228
Methanol, 99+%	nt	nt	80	18.2	>480	nd	nt	nt
2-Methoxy ethanol	nt	nt	nt	nt	nt	nt	nt	nt
2-Methoxyethyl acetate, 98%	nt	nt	260	0.18	nt	nt	nt	nt
Methyl bromide	nt	nt	47	0.000047	nt	nt	nt	nt
Methyl ethyl ketone, 99%	nt	nt	29	1.3	nt	nt	nt	nt
Methyl isocyanate	nt	nt	2	35	nt	nt	nt	nt
*Methyl parathion, 57%	15	0.015	120-180	0.0017	nt	nt	nt	nt
*Methyl parathion, 10%	30-45	0.033	>240	<0.0003	nt	nt	nt	nt
Methylene chloride, 99+%	<1	99.5	80	53	10	26	>299	0.0058

nd = none detected   nm = not measured   nt = not tested

*Chemicals marked with an asterisk may require a Level A, gas-tight suit. Suits of TYVEK, TYVEK QC, and TYVEK/Saranex-23P should not be used where gas-tight suits are required.
TYVEK, TYVEK QC, TYVEK/Saranex-23P and BARRICADE should not be used around heat, flame, sparks or in potentially flammable or explosive atmospheres.
This guide replaces all previously published guides and is valid until May 1990. Permeation guides are revised yearly. Call (800) 44-TYVEK for updated guides.

Chemical permeation data

Chemical challenge	TYVEK® QC Coated with 1.25 mil Polyethylene — Breakthrough Time (min.)	Permeation Rate (mg/m²/sec.)	TYVEK® SARANEX®-23P Single Ply — Breakthrough Time (min.)	Permeation Rate (mg/m²/sec.)	TYVEK® SARANEX®-23P Two Ply — Breakthrough Time (min.)	Permeation Rate (mg/m²/sec.)	BARRICADE® — Breakthrough Time (min.)	Permeation Rate (mg/m²/sec.)
Mineral spirits	<5	1.167	>480	nd	nt	nd	>480	nd
*Nitrobenzene, 99%	<15	.333	165	0.1	>480	nt	nt	nd
Nitrogen dioxide gas, 99%	nt	nt	>480	nd	nt	nt	nt	nd
Nitrogen tetroxide	nt	nt	nt	nt	nt	nt	24	10.95
Nitromethane, 98.1%	nt	nt	nt	nt	nt	nt	>480	nd
*Phenol, 99+%	nt	nt	nt	nt	nt	nt	>480	nd
*PCB	nt	nt	nt	nt	nt	nt	>480	nd
*50% PCB, 50% trichlorobenzene	nt	nt	nt	nt	nt	nt	nt	nt
*4% PCB, 6% trichlorobenzene, 90% mineral spirits	nt	nt	nt	nt	nt	nt	nt	nt
*50% PCB, 50% mineral oil	nt	nt	60-120 (PCB)	0.00003	nt	nt	nt	nt
*1% PCB, 99% mineral oil	nt	nt	>480	nd	nt	nt	nt	nt
Sodium dichromate, 3%	>480	nd	>480	nd	nt	nt	nt	nt
Sodium hydroxide, 40%	>480	nd	>480	nd	nt	nt	nt	nt
Sodium hydroxide, 50%	nt	nt	nt	nt	>480	nt	nt	nt
Sodium hydroxide, 99.9%	>480	nd	nt	nt	nt	nt	>480	nd
Sodium hypochlorite, 5.25%	>480	nd	>480	nd	nt	nt	>480	nd
Styrene, 99%	nt	nt	43	11.6	nt	nt	>480	nd
Sulfuric acid, 95+%	>480	nd	>480	nd	>480	nt	>480	nd
Sulfur dioxide	nt	nt	nt	nt	nt	nt	>480	nd
Tetrachloroethane, 98%	nt	nt	75	2	nt	nt	nt	nt
Tetrachloroethylene, 99%	1	68.347	13	0.19	303	2	>480	nd
Tetrahydrofuran 99%	nt	nt	12	nt	12	21	>480	nd
Toluene, 98+%	<1	30.5561	<5	3.33	82	8	>480	nd
Toluene diisocyanate, 80%	immed.	7	>480	nd	nt	nt	>480	nd
o-Toluidine	<15	0.167	>120	<0.005	nt	nt	nt	nt
Trichlorobenzene	<15	0.833	15-60	<0.0167	nt	nt	>480	nd
1,1,1-Trichloroethane, 97%	nt	nt	nt	nt	nt	nt	nt	nt
2,2,2-Trichloroethanol, 98%	nt	nt	19	2.2	nt	nt	nt	nt
Triethylamine, 99%	nt	nt	>480	nd	nt	nt	nt	nt
2,2,2-Trifluoroethanol, 99%	nm	nm	nt	nt	nt	nt	nt	nt
Xylene	6	nm	nt	nt	nt	nt	>480	nd

nd = none detected   nm = not measured   nt = not tested

*Chemicals marked with an asterisk may require a Level A, gas-tight suit. Suits of TYVEK, TYVEK QC, and TYVEK/Saranex-23P should not be used where gas-tight suits are required.
TYVEK, TYVEK QC, TYVEK/Saranex-23P and BARRICADE should not be used around heat, flame, sparks or in potentially flammable or explosive atmospheres.
This guide replaces all previously published guides and is valid until May 1990. Permeation guides are revised yearly. Call (800) 44-TYVEK for updated guides.

Figure 7-6 (*continued*)

Ease of Decontamination

After use, CPC must be decontaminated. It is not always possible to remove a contaminating chemical from CPC completely. This is due in part to the ability of chemicals to permeate the material and remain within the suit material (see later discussion). No assurance exists that a suit exposed to high concentrations of a hazardous chemical will maintain its chemical resistance. For this reason, disposable CPC may be preferable to reusable suits.

Temperature Resistance

The resistance of suit materials is usually determined at room temperature. These materials may provide different resistance and protection at higher or lower temperatures. Moreover, suits may become stiff and difficult to use at high or low ambient temperatures. Before selecting CPC material, services should consider the climate in which it will most often be used. Responders must also recognize that CPC does not provide protection against heat or fire. High-temperature clothing, such as proximity suits and fire entry suits, are highly specialized and expensive equipment that have no likely value to EMS personnel. A proximity suit is illustrated in Figure 7–7. A fully encapsulating Level A suit with flash protection is illustrated in Figure 7–8.

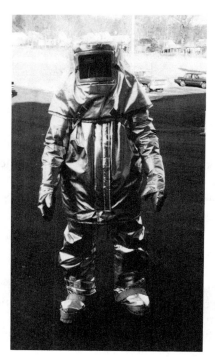

Figure 7–7 Typical proximity suit providing protection from radiant heat and high temperatures. This garment should not be used for entry into fire or direct flame contact.

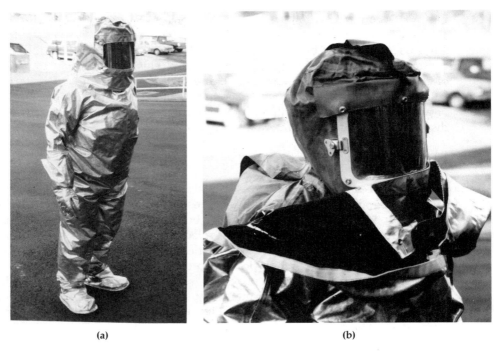

(a)   **(b)**

Figure 7–8   (a) Level A butyl protective ensemble with aluminized NOMEX®
outer covering. The internal Level A protection is provided for high chemical
toxicity or corrosivity, and the aluminized NOMEX® outer garment is protection
from a flash fire or ignition of gaseous vapors. (b) Illustration of the butyl Level
A protection inside and NOMEX-flash protection outside. (NOMEX® produced
by Du Pont, Wilmington, DE).

Cost

An enormous price difference exists between disposable nonencapsulating suits
and technically sophisticated reusable ensembles. Response services should
carefully consider the actual uses that they will make of CPC before buying expensive equipment.

CHEMICAL RESISTANCE

Chemical protective clothing is used as a shield to keep harmful chemicals away
from responders working in contaminated areas. Such chemicals can enter CPC
as a result of penetration, degradation, and permeation. The material from
which CPC is made and the integrity of the CPC determine the effectiveness of
that shield.

Penetration is the process by which chemicals enter a suit through openings in the garment. A chemical can penetrate through stitched seams, button holes, pinholes, zippers, and between the threads of a woven fabric. Rips, tears, punctures, or abrasions of the garment material can also allow penetration. To prevent chemical penetration, CPC uses self-sealing zippers, seams overlaid with tape, flap closures, and nonwoven fabrics.

Degradation refers to the actions of chemicals, heat, and light on the CPC suit material, which lead to material breakdown and damage. As a result of degradation, the material loses its ability to resist chemical entry. Signs of fabric degradation include shrinking, swelling, brittleness, cracking, discoloration, and stickiness.

Permeation is the process by which molecules of a chemical diffuse through the CPC material. Permeation does not injure or damage the material and does not cause changes that are visually obvious. Virtually every material used for CPC allows some permeation by some chemicals. Once a chemical has begun to permeate, no assurance exists that it can be removed during decontamination.

Chemical resistance of fabrics and materials can be measured by standardized laboratory methods. The ability of chemicals to degrade CPC fabrics and materials is routinely measured by exposing pieces of the fabric to chemicals for fixed time periods. This approach is often used to develop chemical compatibility charts that are frequently the basis for choosing CPC.

Permeation by chemicals is measured by applying standard volumes of chemicals to one side of a fabric, and then evaluating the speed of permeation and the quantity that permeates over time. The elapsed time between the application of a chemical to a protective material's outer surface and its initial appearance at the inner surface is the *breakthrough time*. The *permeation rate* is a measure of the quantity of chemical that permeates a given area of material in a given time.

In choosing a protective material, a long breakthrough time and low permeation rate are desirable. Responders must remember, however, that these measures are usually made under standard conditions, and materials may act differently as conditions change. For example, permeation increases as temperatures rise. Also, mixtures of chemicals can permeate more quickly than do the individual chemicals alone. Likewise, degradation of CPC material occurs more quickly as temperatures increase and after exposure to chemical mixtures.

SELECTION OF CHEMICAL PROTECTIVE CLOTHING BY EMERGENCY MEDICAL SERVICES PERSONNEL

Most EMS personnel will never be asked to enter areas of high-level hazardous material contamination. Entry into such areas will usually be restricted to specially trained hazardous materials teams and fire service personnel. For that reason, it is unlikely that most emergency medical technicians or paramedics will ever actually work in fully encapsulating Level A suits. Moreover, few EMS skills can be carried out by a technician wearing CPC equipment. For example, a stethoscope cannot be used by a responder in a fully encapsulating suit. Likewise, a rescuer wearing double-layered, chemical resistant gloves can neither feel a pulse nor manipulate an intravenous setup.

Nevertheless, it is possible to imagine situations in which entry by EMS personnel may be desirable. The proper role for EMS responders in such situations remains controversial. For example, EMS personnel may be asked to perform field triage and assessment of victims within the contaminated zone at hazardous materials incidents with many casualties. Or EMS responders may be asked to provide care to victims trapped by debris who cannot be immediately extricated from a contaminated area.

For such reasons, EMS personnel should receive training to be at least familiar with the design and use of Level A equipment. They should also be familiar with procedures and policies necessary to assure their own safety. Protection of EMS responders and other health care workers is discussed in more detail in chapter 14.

Even if EMS personnel do not enter the hot zones of hazardous materials incidents, they will risk some exposure when they care for incident victims. Those victims may suffer low-level contamination despite having undergone decontamination. Personnel who are in contact with such victims may become contaminated. This might include victims of acid or alkali splashes, those exposed to insecticides, toxic dusts, and toxic gases.

To protect against contamination in such situations, EMS and other health care personnel may benefit from the use of disposable, nonencapsulating, Level B clothing. Disposable CPC made of Tyvek, particularly when coated with either polyethylene or Saranex, or stand-alone materials such as Barricade and Chemrel can protect against splash exposures owing to many liquid chemicals as well as exposures to toxic dusts and powders. Multiple layers of gloves can prevent hand exposure without restricting the movements and dexterity necessary to perform EMS and health care procedures. The use of inexpensive, disposable outfits allows EMS personnel and other health care providers to avoid the need for CPC decontamination. A more extensive discussion of methods for preventing contamination of the EMS and health care systems is presented in chapter 14.

SUMMARY

Chemical protective equipment includes respiratory protection and chemical protective clothing. The choice of each depends on the chemicals that are present at an incident, their concentrations, and their likely routes of exposure. Air supply devices should be used for respiratory protection except when the chemical has been identified and is known to be present in concentrations for which air purification respirators can be safely used.

Protective clothing is available in various designs and fabrics that provide several different levels of protection. For exposure to IDLH environments or for prolonged exposure to chemicals toxic by skin contact, fully encapsulating Level A suits should be worn. For lower levels of exposure, nonencapsulating Level B protection may be adequate. The actual choice of suit material and design must be based on the chemical compatibility and permeability characteristics of the individual suits that are available.

EMS personnel and other health care providers who are likely to be at risk of hazardous materials contamination should be trained in the use of personal protective equipment. Those personnel who may be in contact with incompletely decontaminated victims outside of the zone of high contamination should consider wearing disposable, nonencapsulating, Level B protective suits and at least double layers of surgical gloves. They should also be familiar with the design and use of fully encapsulating Level A suits, although they are unlikely to need such high levels of protection.

REFERENCES

CARLSON, GENE P., ed., *HazMat Response Team Leak and Spill Guide.* Stillwater, Okla.: Fire Protection Publications, Oklahoma State University, 1984.

''Hazardous Waste Operations and Emergency Response: Notice of Proposed Rulemaking and Public Hearings,'' Department of Labor, OSHA, 29 CFR Part 1910. *Federal Register,* 54, no. 42 (March 6, 1989), p. 9294–9336.

NIOSH Respirator Decision Logic: U.S. Department of Health and Human Services, May 1987.

Occupational Safety and Health Guidance Manual for Hazardous Waste Site Activities: U.S. Department of Health and Human Services, October 1985.

PLANNING THE EMERGENCY MEDICAL SERVICES RESPONSE

CHAPTER 8

GOAL: On completion of this chapter the student will be able to describe the kinds of information that must be gathered and the important planning decisions to be made before a rescue can occur.

OBJECTIVES:

Specifically, the student will be able to

- Discuss the information needed to assure that a rescue can be carried out safely
- Name the three types of emergency situations into which hazardous materials incidents can be categorized
- Discuss the importance of the buddy system

OVERVIEW

EMS personnel are usually action-oriented people who are eager to help. Because they want to be involved and are trained to provide care quickly, standing by or delaying help for the sick or injured can be difficult for them. Moreover, it is standard teaching that successful EMS operations generally demand quick response and rapid intervention. This is especially true when care is provided to victims of severe trauma and critical illness.

Certain kinds of incidents, however, require a slow and deliberate EMS response. Responders may have no choice but to stand by and watch or wait until the situation allows them to become involved. This occurs most often at fire scenes. EMS personnel are usually not allowed to enter burning buildings and must wait for victims to be brought out before care can be given.

In such situations, the guiding principle is that the EMS responders must not expose themselves to unnecessary risks. Little is gained, and much is lost at an accident scene if emergency responders and rescuers become victims.

This principle must also be applied to hazardous materials incidents. Rescuers must take special precautions to avoid being contaminated or injured by hazardous chemicals. As a result, the EMS response must be begun deliberately and systematically. It is necessary to gather information and plan the rescue carefully before any patient care can be given.

In this chapter, we will consider the kinds of information that must be gathered and the important planning decisions to be made before EMS personnel can safely carry out victim rescue at a hazardous materials incident.

INFORMATION GATHERING

Before beginning the rescue and emergency care of victims, EMS rescuers must determine whether a hazardous materials incident exists, whether it poses a risk to them or the victims, and whether they can safely carry out their EMS functions. The following information is needed to assure that a rescue can be carried out safely:

1. Is a hazardous material present?

2. Does the hazard pose a risk to the rescue team?

3. Can the risk be reduced to permit a rescue?

4. Is the rescue team prepared?

Is a hazardous material present?   It is not always obvious that an incident involves hazardous materials. Fortunately, in most cases that information will be immediately available and provided to EMS responders at the time that they are dispatched to the scene. In other situations, however, the presence of a hazardous chemical may be a surprise. Such surprises are rarely pleasant.

EMS teams should not be surprised by the presence of industrial hazards when responding to accidents at large chemical plants or factories. Those are locations at which we expect to find chemical hazards. In almost every case, plant employees know about those hazards and can provide needed information to responders. In addition, most industrial users of hazardous chemicals are required by SARA to submit lists of their hazardous chemicals to local emergency planning committees.

Conversely, hazardous surprises may be found where chemicals are used or stored in home laboratories, garages, small warehouses, and at noncomplying manufacturers.

Similarly, large transport tankers and railroad cars filled with hazardous chemicals usually carry proper placards and documentation. They allow emergency responders to recognize the presence and identity of hazardous materials easily following transportation accidents. Small but potentially harmful quantities of chemicals, however, are often shipped without placards in trucks and private cars. In those cases, vehicular accidents can result in unexpected hazardous materials incidents.

EMS responders must always consider the possibility of hazardous materials to avoid becoming victims.

Does the hazard pose a risk to rescuers?   The known presence of a hazard does not necessarily mean that it poses risks to victims or rescuers. For example, a gas may reach high concentrations in a closed, unventilated room and injure trapped victims. Once the room has been ventilated, however, the concentration can quickly fall to harmless levels. Before ventilation, rescuers cannot enter because of the dangerous concentrations that would threaten them. Following ventilation, rescuers can enter and provide emergency care without fear of being harmed.

Likewise, some flammable gases form explosive mixtures with air, but only at temperatures that are higher than normal room temperature. In a room that is cooler than normal, those gases pose little fire or explosion risk. Rescuers can safely enter and care for victims as the room temperature remains well below the ignition temperature of the chemical involved. If that room temperature becomes elevated and approaches the degree at which those gases can explode, however, then rescuers face great risk by entering.

Once the presence of a hazardous chemical has been confirmed, EMS responders must decide whether that material poses a risk to them. This requires identifying the material and determining the amount that is present.

The actual identification and measurement of chemicals present is usually carried out by fire service personnel. It is possible in some situations that EMS personnel will need to perform these identification and measurement tasks. It is essential that the identity and exposure risks of hazardous materials be established before EMS rescuers enter a contaminated place. EMS personnel should not enter such a place if there is a likely risk of injury.

Can the risk be reduced enough to permit a rescue?   It is sometimes possible to reduce the risk posed by hazards for safe rescue of victims by EMS personnel. This can be done by using environmental controls that decrease the risks of the contaminated place. It can also be achieved by providing special protection to the rescuers.

The use of environmental controls can serve to reduce contamination to safe levels. For example, ventilating a contaminated closed space can greatly decrease the concentration of a hazardous gas. The use of water sprays and mists can remove large amounts of water soluble gases from the air and make safe entry possible.

The decision to use environmental controls is rarely the responsibility of EMS personnel. It is usually a decision made by fire service officers. Before entry, EMS teams must assure themselves that the use of such controls has successfully reduced exposure risks.

The use of personal protective equipment is another approach to reducing risks to rescuers. Although heavy gloves, fully encapsulating suits, and SCBA face masks make difficult many of the diagnostic and assessment tasks, rescuers are able to gain access to victims. Rapid extrication of those victims can be safely completed. Once victims have been moved to safe locations outside the contaminated area, emergency medical care can be provided without danger to the EMS team.

Is the rescue team prepared?   EMS personnel should understand the basic concepts of hazardous materials management. Earlier we have addressed issues and skills that are often regarded as ''fire service skills.'' EMS services, however, will often be involved in caring for the victims of hazardous materials accidents. Members of those EMS services are likely to risk exposure at such accidents. Therefore, those chapters also describe ''EMS skills.'' To protect themselves, EMS personnel must be knowledgeable about hazardous materials.

EMS responders who lack understanding of hazardous materials are not prepared to care for the victims of hazardous materials exposure. Similarly, EMS personnel who lack understanding of the use of personal protective equipment cannot safely respond to large hazardous materials incidents.

Conversely, EMS team members can learn the basic concepts of hazardous materials response and the advantages of different kinds of protective equipment. EMS personnel can then participate fully in planning and performing the safe rescues of hazardous materials victims.

RESCUE PLANNING

On the basis of the information that has been gathered, EMS responders can categorize hazardous materials incidents into three types of emergency situations. For each, a different set of safety concerns and possible emergency responses exists. The job of planning the rescue involves first determining which type of emergency situation exists and the possible responses.

In one type of emergency situation, no EMS response is possible. For example, in some emergencies neither environmental controls nor protective equipment can make the situation safe. A second situation occurs when rescuers can safely ignore the hazardous material and carry out a normal EMS response. Between those two situations are cases in which a modified EMS response, generally based on rapid extrication of victims, can be completed.

No Response

Some hazardous materials incidents pose such great risk to responders that rescue efforts are not possible or must be delayed. EMS responders should not enter environments that pose great threat to them. One example involves an environment contaminated by a flammable and explosive gas where the environmental temperature is at or above the chemical's ignition temperature. In this case, the threat of explosion may be so great that all rescuers must stay at a distance.

Another example occurs when an environment is contaminated by high concentrations of a lethal chemical and responders do not have appropriate protective equipment. Entry into the contaminated area by unprotected rescuers is dangerous to the rescuers.

In these settings, rescuers must determine that an IDLH environment exists from which they cannot be protected. This is similar to fire situations in which EMS responders do not enter because of the dangers that are present.

These are among the most difficult and frustrating situations that confront emergency medical technicians and paramedics because they can do nothing while victims suffer or die. Such frustration, however, is preferable to the EMS personnel becoming victims or casualties.

Normal Response

At the other extreme are situations in which EMS personnel responding to hazardous materials victims can disregard the threat to themselves.

An example of such a situation is when a hazardous gas has leaked into a closed, unventilated space, causing injury and harm to trapped victims. Once ventilation has decreased gas concentration to harmless levels, rescuers can safely treat victims by conventional EMS methods.

Another example involves a flammable and explosive gas leaking into a room that has a temperature well below the ignition temperature of that gas. Because little risk of explosion or fire exists, a normal EMS response may be possible.

An EMS response is also appropriate for victims who have been splashed by corrosive chemicals if prompt and thorough skin washing has occurred. Responders must be careful to avoid being contaminated with the chemical on a victim's skin but are otherwise generally safe from chemical harm.

Before EMS providers carry out such "routine" rescues of hazardous chemical victims, they must be certain of a safe environment. In particular, they must be certain of safe chemical concentration levels, sufficient oxygen within closed spaces, and no uncontrolled risks of fire or explosion. If these conditions are unassured, then rescuers should not perform rescues without protective equipment and support.

Modified Response

Finally, situations exist in which EMS responders can spend only brief amounts of time in the contaminated area, or require that protective clothing and equipment be used. Because of the short time available and limitations imposed by protective clothing and equipment, only a modified EMS response can be implemented.

Victims may be found exposed to concentrations of toxic chemicals that do not reach the IDLH level but do exceed the STEL level. The STEL is the concentration that is safe for exposures of less than 15 minutes. Rescuers without protection can safely approach victims, but must spend less than 15 minutes total time in the area of contamination. This limited time span will rarely permit a full assessment of victims, initiation of emergency care, and transport of victims from contamination.

These patients, many of whom may be unconscious or may appear to have suffered trauma, need careful and thorough assessment. Like all other unconscious patients and trauma victims, transport should not be undertaken without full immobilization.

In such situations, rescuers should perform rapid extrication to move victims as rapidly as can be safely done from the area of contamination. Complete assessments can then be carried out in a safer, less contaminated place.

It may sometimes be necessary for EMS personnel to spend more prolonged periods in highly contaminated locations. For example, injured victims may be trapped under fallen debris and require complicated extrication. Multiple casualty situations may occur that demand assessment and prioritization before rescue can be completed. For such settings, responders may need to wear protective clothing and SCBA.

It is not possible, however, to carry out most routine EMS procedures while wearing such equipment. A stethoscope cannot be used by a paramedic wearing a fully encapsulating entry suit. Likewise, heavy protective gloves greatly limit the EMT's ability to feel for wounds and deformities. Accordingly, the assessment phase of the EMS response must be modified as described in chapter 10. In these situations rapid extrication is performed so that victims are quickly and safely moved to a safer place for full assessment.

A modified EMS response involving use of rapid extrication may also be indicated for victims of chemical exposures requiring prompt administration of antidotes not available at the incident site. Exposure to cyanide or hydrogen sulfide are two examples of poisonings that often require almost immediate antidotal treatment to prevent fatality. In such cases, standard assessments and treatment may need to be delayed.

USE OF BUDDY SYSTEM

When activities are to be performed in any area of potential danger, the "buddy system" should be initiated. This concept of cooperation involves the use of two or more emergency responders who enter the dangerous area and work there together. Before EMS personnel enter contaminated places to effect a rescue, they should establish a buddy system.

Use of this multiple person operational approach affords safety for involved emergency personnel. The benefits of the approach include the following:

1. Personnel can assist one another

2. Personnel can observe their buddies' actions to assure the safety of their procedures

3. Personnel can watch each other for signs of fatigue, overexposure, equipment failure, or distress

4. Personnel can monitor the integrity of the protective clothing and equipment used by their buddies

5. Personnel can call for help if their buddies experience trouble or distress

An extension of the buddy system involves the use of dedicated personnel to stand by while others are in the contaminated zone of an incident. This backup group can provide a fresh team to continue operations, or rescue the victim and rescuers, if an accident occurs.

SUMMARY

EMS responders must approach hazardous materials victims in a cautious and thoughtful manner. Before becoming involved in rescue efforts, the nature of the incident and the risks confronting both victims and rescuers must be established. EMS personnel must become familiar with some procedures and information that are often viewed as the primary concern of the fire service.

With appropriate information, EMS personnel can develop rescue plans that consider the needs of both victims and rescuers. In some situations it is not possible to perform a rescue because of the risks to the EMS team. In others, a modified response is appropriate. Without first gathering necessary information, responders risk chemical exposure and injury. It is never appropriate for rescuers to become victims.

MECHANISMS OF HAZARDOUS MATERIALS EXPOSURE AND INJURY

CHAPTER 9

GOAL: On completion of this chapter the student will have an understanding of the routes by which victims can be exposed to hazardous materials and will be able to describe the mechanisms by which those hazardous materials can cause tissue injury.

OBJECTIVES:

Specifically, the student will be able to

- List four routes of exposure by which hazardous materials can cause toxic injury
- Describe hazardous materials incidents leading to exposure by each of the four routes of exposure and by combinations of several of those exposure routes
- List five mechanisms by which hazardous materials can cause tissue injury
- Describe the effects of each of the five mechanisms of injury and provide examples of specific chemicals that can cause those effects

OVERVIEW

Emergency responders must be prepared to care for the victims of chemical exposure even when they know little about the specific chemical causing the emergency. Because so many hazardous chemicals are used in our world, few of us can recognize all of their names. It would be even more difficult to try to remember the ways that each causes injury.

Lack of information about specific chemicals makes the responder's job more difficult. Fortunately, that job is not impossible. Appropriate emergency care can often be provided when only a small amount of information is available. In many cases, the injuries that victims suffer can be predicted by knowing only the class or type of chemical involved.

To anticipate the harmful effects of a chemical exposure, rescuers must know the various ways that chemicals cause damage. In this chapter, the routes of exposure that lead to toxic injury and some of the mechanisms by which chemicals cause harm are considered. Following chapters present in greater detail the clinical effects of chemicals on the lungs (chapter 15), the eyes (chapter 16), the skin (chapter 17), and after systemic absorption (chapter 18).

ROUTES OF EXPOSURE

Four routes of exposure to hazardous chemicals include the following:

1. Inhalation

2. Skin

3. Eye

4. Ingestion

Some victims become exposed by only a single route. A worker, for example, may splash acid on his skin but not suffer eye contact or inhalation exposure. In other cases, exposures involve two or more routes. Victims exposed to high concentrations of irritating gases, such as ammonia and chlorine, can suffer injury as a result of skin contact, eye contact, and inhalation.

The assessment of a victim must include careful consideration of all possible exposure routes. Otherwise, some injuries may go unnoticed and proper care will be delayed. Inhalation exposure can occur when a chemical is splashed on the chest, shoulders, or face. Unless suspected, it may not be recognized until severe lung injury has developed. Likewise, the signs of skin exposure may not be obvious. Skin absorption of small amounts of some chemicals (such as cyanide), however, can produce lethal effects and require urgent care.

Inhalation

We inhale toxic chemicals, usually in small quantities, with almost every breath we take. The harmful effects of cigarette smoke and air pollution are well known. Such toxic inhalations occur chronically and produce slowly developing damage. Inhalation of immediately harmful quantities of hazardous chemicals can result from industrial accidents, transportation accidents, and fires. Smoke inhalation is a commonly encountered type of toxic exposure. Similar injury can result from exposure to a wide assortment of toxic gases, mists, and dusts.

The lungs are particularly vulnerable to exposure injuries because of their structure. The alveoli, for example, consist of a large surface of thin, unprotected membrane. In an average person, the alveolar surface area is about as large as a tennis court. Such a huge surface is ideal for the lungs' normal function of exchanging oxygen and carbon dioxide. It also permits rapid absorption of inhaled toxic gases, however.

In addition, irritant gases can easily injure alveoli. Strong irritants, such as ammonia or chlorine, burn the alveolar membranes in the same way that they burn the skin. Because the alveolar surface area is so much greater than the skin's, however, inhalation burns can cause more injury than total body skin burns.

The body has defenses to protect against inhalation exposure. At rest, most inhaled air passes through the nose where fine hairs and cilia remove potentially toxic dust particles and mist droplets. Many inhaled chemicals also dissolve in the moisture coating the mucous membranes in the nose and pharynx. Chemicals are trapped by airway mucus before reaching the alveoli. In these ways, many contaminants are removed before air enters the alveoli.

During industrial accidents and chemical releases, however, these protective mechanisms may fail. This can happen for the following reasons:

1. The quantity of toxic chemicals in inhaled air may be so great that only a small proportion can be removed before the air reaches the lungs.
2. People who are injured, frightened, or performing hard work breathe through the mouth instead of the nose. Mouth breathing is much less effective in removing chemicals from inhaled air. Therefore, victims and rescuers are more likely to suffer inhalation exposure.
3. The volume of air inhaled each minute increases when people are frightened or working hard. During strenuous exercise, the inhaled air volume can be twenty times greater than at rest. Increasing the volume of inhaled air leads to a greater quantity of airborne chemicals drawn into the lungs. The amount of those chemicals that are absorbed also increases.

Inhalation exposure must be considered in every hazardous materials victim. Assessment of the lungs, including evaluation of respiratory pattern and lung sounds, is important. The onset of severe lung disorders, such as pulmonary edema and asthma, can be delayed for hours after exposure. Therefore, inhalation victims and those suspected of inhalation exposure must be reassessed periodically.

Skin

Toxic skin exposure can result from liquids that splash or spill as well as contact with gases, mists, and dusts. Reactive chemicals, such as strong acids and alkali, can cause rapid injury that is immediately obvious. Other chemicals cause delayed damage or death but produce few early signs. Unlike thermal skin burns, the severity of chemical burns cannot usually be determined during the first 24 to 48 hours.

Many chemicals can be absorbed from the skin and cause systemic poisoning. Some, such as hydrogen cyanide, can be fatal to victims after only a tiny amount is absorbed. Such agents may cause only minor skin damage, and skin exposure may not be appreciated until serious toxic effects have developed.

It is important to determine whether skin exposure has occurred. This may require a search for clues such as wet spots on an exposed worker's clothing.

Eye

The eye is extremely sensitive to the effects of chemicals. Commonly encountered examples include the irritation that results from an evening spent in a smoke-filled room, the tear gas–like effects of freshly chopped onions, and the intense pain caused by soaps and shampoos.

The most dangerous injuries result from reactive chemicals that splash into the eye. Such exposures to concentrated alkali or acids can rapidly lead to blindness. Irritant gases can also cause severe eye injuries. In general, gases that cause inhalation injury also damage the eye. Ocular toxicity can occur, however, at air concentrations too low to cause significant lung damage.

It is rarely possible to judge the severity of a chemical eye injury until 24 or more hours after exposure. At first, few differences exist between the appearance of a mildly damaged eye and one that has suffered devastating exposure. Because the eyes are so sensitive and can quickly suffer damage, prompt recognition of exposure is important. Following splashes to the face or exposure to irritating gases, victims should be managed as though eye exposure had occurred.

Ingestion

Most toxic chemicals cause serious injury when swallowed. Severe burns of the mouth, esophagus, and stomach can result from many ingested chemicals. Absorption of others can lead to systemic poisoning. Because larger quantities of chemicals can be swallowed than are absorbed from the lungs or skin, ingestion poisonings are often severer than other exposures.

Ingestion exposures are rarely the result of industrial accidents. Infrequently, community food or water supplies are contaminated by such accidents. Eating or drinking that food or water can then cause medical emergencies. After inhalation exposure, small amounts of chemical may mix with sputum and saliva and be swallowed.

Emergency response personnel risk ingestion exposure when they fail to undergo proper decontamination. For example, if a rescuer eats food or smokes a cigarette while his or her hands are still contaminated, then it is likely that the contaminant will be carried into that rescuer's mouth and swallowed. Response personnel must be careful to avoid such exposures.

Generally ingestion exposures result from suicide attempts and childhood accidents. Because the focus of this book is the health effects of industrial accidents, ingestion exposures will not be further considered.

MECHANISMS OF INJURY

Toxic chemicals injure by interfering with the normal functions and activities of the body's cells. In some cases, the mechanism of chemical injury is precise. The lethal effects of hydrogen cyanide, for example, are due to disruption of a single enzyme, cytochrome oxidase. In other cases, the combined effects of several mechanisms of injury damage cells in a nonselective way and cause massive tissue destruction. Strong acids and alkali produce harm in this way.

The mechanisms by which chemicals produce injury can be categorized into at least the following groups:

1. Thermal injury: cold
2. Thermal injury: heat
3. Mechanical injury
4. Ischemic injury
5. Chemical reactions
   - Nonselective injury corrosives
   - Selective injury chemicals

Thermal Injury: Cold

Many chemicals that normally exist as gases are stored as compressed gases, as liquified gases, or as extremely cold cryogenic gases. When compressed or liquified gases are released, they expand violently and become very cold. This is the principle by which most modern refrigerators operate. Contact with such gases as they leak from a tank or cylinder causes freeze injury of exposed body surfaces. Severer freeze damage results from contact with cryogenic gases that may be more than 100° colder than the freezing point of water.

Thermal Injury: Heat

Thermal burns can result from chemical exposure. More than 65 percent of hazardous chemicals are flammable liquids that pose risks of fire when released. Once ignited, explosive fires can result that burn victims and rescuers.

Nonflammable chemicals can also cause thermal burns. Some react with water to yield large amounts of heat. Chemical reactions that produce heat are called *exothermic reactions*. Because water is present throughout the body, exothermic reactions can occur from body contact with chemicals of this sort. Thermal burns of exposed skin, eye, or lung may result. Chemicals that produce thermal burns in this way include sulfuric acid, ammonia, and active metals such as sodium.

Mechanical Injury

Some chemicals produce "mechanical" injury leading to tissue damage and cell death. Violent dehydration of cells can be caused by chemicals that have extremely strong attraction for water. Sulfuric acid causes this kind of injury.

Another type of mechanical injury results from gases that displace oxygen in the atmosphere and cause asphyxiation. Oxygen-poor environments can occur when pressurized gas is forced into a closed tank car or unventilated room. People who enter those spaces can be quickly overcome. Inhalation of heavier-than-air gases can prevent oxygen-containing air from entering the lungs.

Ischemic Injury

Chemicals that provoke intense inflammation can damage the blood vessels of affected tissues. Vascular thrombosis and occlusion, decreased blood flow, and ischemia of involved tissues can result. Vascular thromboses occur in the lungs, skin, and eyes of victims exposed to acids, alkali, and other reactive chemicals. Ischemia of the cornea after alkali burns usually leads to blindness and eye loss.

Chemical Reaction

Most hazardous chemicals cause injury by reacting with body tissues to alter the structure or function of cells and their components.

In some cases, damage results from violent reactions that disrupt many cellular functions and destroy many types of cells. The injuries caused by strong corrosives such as acids and alkali are examples.

In other cases, chemicals have precise toxic effects interfering with only a few specific proteins or enzymes. Hydrogen cyanide, which causes death by blocking the functions of a single enzyme, cytochrome oxidase, is an example of such a chemical.

Examples of the injurious reactions caused by some common groups of industrial chemicals are listed subsequently.

Nonselective injury corrosives.   These corrosives cause massive destruction to the substance of tissues. Many chemicals (including most acids, alkali, and amines) act as corrosives. In addition to causing thermal burns, mechanical injury, and ischemia, corrosives react chemically with proteins, fats, and other tissue structures.

Acids cause proteins to precipitate as a dense, clotlike "coagulum" that covers the injured area. This destructive process of acids is known as *coagulation necrosis*. Once formed, the coagulum provides protection against further injury by absorbing and neutralizing some of the acid and by blocking deep penetration.

Alkali dissolve fats and lipids from cell membranes and cause the cells to fall apart. Solid tissue is changed into a soapy liquid by a process called *liquefaction necrosis*. Alkali also disrupt and destroy proteins and other essential components of tissue. Unlike acid-induced coagulation necrosis, liquefaction necrosis does not block deep penetration by alkali. For that reason, alkali burns can be much deeper and more destructive than acid burns.

Vesicants and *alkylating agents* are reactive chemicals that bind to and disrupt proteins, deoxyribonucleic acid (DNA), and other macromolecules. Many of the poison gases used during World War I, such as mustard gas and Lewisite, were vesicants or alkylating agents. At high concentrations vesicants cause severe blistering. At low concentrations they act like tear gas. Large areas of the skin and lung membranes can be destroyed by high-concentration exposure. Alkylating agents can cause severe, acute injury to many body systems. Because they can alter cellular DNA, many alkylating agents are regarded as potential causes of cancer after long-term exposure.

Selective injury chemicals. Some chemicals produce devastating injury or death by causing precise disturbances in cellular function. These chemicals may inhibit a biologic process or alter the concentrations of specific salts in the blood.

Enzyme poisons are chemicals that inhibit cellular reactions that are often essential for survival. Most enzymes are proteins that enable or accelerate chemical reactions. Cellular use of oxygen, for example, depends on a family of enzymes called *cytochrome oxidases*. Poisoning of those enzymes by chemicals such as cyanide or hydrogen sulfide makes cells unable to use oxygen and cellular anoxia develops. Exposure to enzyme poisons can lead to immediate death.

Sequestration agents bind specific salts and make them unavailable to the cells. Calcium, for example, is essential for many cellular functions and may be removed from the blood of exposed victims by hydrogen fluoride or oxalic acid. Low blood calcium concentrations, or *hypocalcemia*, leads to cell death, seizures, and cardiac arrest.

Other *metabolic poisons* cause toxic products to accumulate and produce cell injury. In some cases, harmless chemicals are absorbed and then changed to harmful agents. Methanol, for example, causes ethanol-like intoxication but is not itself a cause of serious damage. It is converted in the body to formic acid, however, which accumulates and causes nervous system injury and blindness.

SUMMARY

Chemicals can cause injury in various ways and after different kinds of exposure. Even when little is known about the specific chemical involved, proper care can often be provided.

A careful assessment of the victim must be performed. It is important to determine the specific routes of exposure that occurred. Failure to recognize all exposure routes may cause injuries to be ignored and delay proper care.

It is often possible to predict the injuries that result from exposure by understanding the ways chemicals cause injury.

ASSESSMENT OF HAZARDOUS MATERIALS VICTIMS

CHAPTER 10

GOAL: On completion of this chapter the student will be able to carry out a proper patient assessment and will understand some specific issues that are of particular importance when managing hazardous materials incidents.

OBJECTIVES:

Specifically, the student will be able to

- Name the four phases of a patient assessment
- Name at least four sources from whom to get information about an incident
- Discuss the information that is pertinent to providing proper patient care
- Discuss the difficulties in relying on victims to provide information
- Name the two phases of an objective examination
- Identify the specific areas to be assessed during the primary survey
- Identify the systemic areas to be assessed during the secondary survey
- Name the components of the secondary survey and discuss specific findings that indicate exposure to hazardous materials
- Describe the formulation of a clinical impression
- Name the goals of a treatment plan

OVERVIEW

This chapter considers the EMS assessment of hazardous materials exposure victims. EMS management and care of these victims is determined on the basis of findings from a careful and accurate assessment. As with all other emergency patients, each victim and his or her injuries must be separately evaluated.

A standard EMS assessment (including subjective interview, objective examination, clinical impression, and treatment plan) should be carried out for each victim. Using a systematic approach, rescuers can usually identify the various effects of exposure even when the hazardous material is one that is unfamiliar.

COMPONENTS OF PATIENT ASSESSMENT

The following four phases should be part of the standard patient assessment of all hazardous materials victims:

1. Subjective interview

2. Objective examination

3. Clinical impression

4. Treatment plan

SUBJECTIVE INTERVIEW

In a hazardous materials emergency, obtaining accurate information about the incident is critical. Usually, the most important source of information is the victim. Other useful sources of information can include bystanders, first responders, plant safety officers, fire department personnel, and co-workers. Information pertinent to providing proper patient care includes the following:

1. What is the toxin?

2. What was the route of exposure (inhalation, ingestion, skin contact)?

3. How large was the exposure dose?

4. How long was the duration of exposure?

5. What other hazardous materials might be present?

6. What are the medical needs of victims exposed to these specific hazardous materials?

The victim is often the person who can best inform rescuers about the nature of the incident; the mechanisms of injury; and medical information such as the victim's past medical history, current medications, allergies, and current chief complaint. Information obtained from exposure victims, however, may be inaccurate because of the effects of toxic chemicals on the central nervous system (CNS).

Many chemicals, such as most organic solvents, cause CNS depression, drowsiness, drunkenness, or stupor. Victims suffering such exposures are unreliable as sources of information because exposure can cause confused thinking and poor memory. Many chemical exposure victims may provide unreliable information for this reason.

Rescuers should obtain as much information as possible about the hazardous material. The identity of the hazardous material and its concentration in the contaminated area must be determined to be certain that rescuers are adequately protected. Without proper protection, rescuers risk exposure and injury. Identification and risk assessment should be made before EMS personnel are allowed to enter the contaminated area and before they have physical contact with contaminated victims. Procedures to protect EMS personnel from contamination are discussed in chapter 14.

OBJECTIVE EXAMINATION

A systematic, hands-on examination of decontaminated patients should be conducted beginning at the head and ending at the feet. The patient's entire body should be included. The objective examination is generally conducted in two phases: the primary survey and the secondary survey.

Primary Survey

The primary survey is an assessment of the vital functions of life. It serves to identify the presence of immediately life-threatening problems. When performing this part of the examination, responders should pay specific attention to assessment of the following:

1. Airway

2. Breathing

3. Circulation

4. Level of consciousness

The *airway assessment* determines whether the airway is open and unobstructed and whether it can be maintained that way. The presence of a gag reflex should be determined. Inhalation of many chemicals—especially reactive, water-soluble ones—can cause rapidly evolving injury of the upper airway that leads to laryngospasm, airway obstruction, and asphyxia. Such chemicals can cause mouth, throat, and nose burns. Therefore, part of the airway assessment of inhalation victims should be a quick but careful search for burns or chemical residue around or inside the mouth and nose.

The *breathing assessment* evaluates a victim's ability to move air into and out of the lungs. Evaluation should be made of the depth, rate, and regularity of breathing. The "look, listen, and feel" method is most commonly used for breathing assessments. Hazardous chemicals can cause a wide variety of breathing disturbances including pulmonary edema, asthma, and respiratory arrest as a result of neurological toxicity. Sometimes these effects are delayed. A careful assessment of breathing as part of the primary assessment should be followed by repeated reassessments. Repeat assessment can lead to earlier recognition of delayed-onset inhalation injury.

The *circulation assessment* determines whether adequate tissue perfusion exists. Effective circulation depends on an efficiently pumping heart, adequate blood volume, and vascular integrity. Measurement of systolic blood pressure and palpation of the carotid artery are generally used to assess the adequacy of the circulation. Other indicators of adequate tissue perfusion include a normal level of consciousness, normal skin color, and the presence of normal arterial pulses. Hypoperfusion and shock can result from exposure to chemicals that cause CNS depression, vascular disturbances, or directly interfere with the heart work and rhythm.

The *level-of-consciousness assessment* can be made by observing the victim's responses to verbal and tactile stimuli. An unconscious victim can lose the gag reflex and the ability to protect the airway. Such patients require close observation and care. These victims may have inadequate circulation and blood pressure.

Secondary Survey

The secondary survey is a systematic patient assessment that determines the presence of injuries or abnormalities that are not immediately life threatening, but that require attention and care. The survey includes a subjective interview and a physical examination carried out mostly by touch. Beginning at the head, the rescuer palpates all body parts as the examination moves down toward the feet.

Some abnormalities (such as gross deformities, ecchymoses, and soft-tissue injuries) may be apparent on visual examination. These findings are important clues to underlying structural damage and require further examination and assessment. During the secondary survey, patients should be checked for medical alert bracelets, tags, and other medical identification devices.

Hazardous materials exposure and trauma often occur together as a result of fires, explosions, accidents at industrial plants, and vehicular accidents involving chemical carriers. Rescuers caring for exposure victims should pay close attention to the possible presence of trauma. Responders caring for unconscious exposure victims should assume that traumatic injuries are present.

The secondary survey is generally divided according to the anatomic regions of the body. The information obtained, however, helps to answer questions of a more general and systematic nature such as the following:

1. Why is the patient unconscious?
2. Why is the patient in respiratory distress?
3. Why is the patient's circulation depressed?
4. Has the patient suffered severe trauma?

Why is the patient unconscious?   Many chemicals can act on the central nervous system and cause depressed consciousness. Some, such as solvents, act like ethanol and cause progressive drunkenness. Others are anesthetics. A few, such as cyanide, are enzyme poisons that block the functions of the body's cells including those in the brain. Interruption of brain cell function can lead to loss of consciousness.

It is difficult to be sure that unconsciousness in an exposure victim is due solely to poisoning. For example, some victims may also have fallen and suffered head trauma. In others, CNS injuries such as strokes or intracranial bleeding may be the reason that consciousness has been lost. The secondary survey helps to discriminate between such alternative possibilities.

Why is the patient in respiratory distress?   Toxic inhalations can effect the respiratory system in many different ways. As described in chapter 15, water soluble chemicals (such as chlorine and ammonia) can cause intense inflammation of the upper airway. Laryngospasm and airway obstruction can result. Other less soluble gases (such as phosgene) act at the alveolar level and produce pulmonary edema. Asphyxiants (such as carbon dioxide and methane) displace oxygen, whereas others (such as cyanide and hydrogen sulfide) block the respiratory functions of cells.

A careful assessment helps to determine the type of respiratory injury that an exposure victim has suffered. Upper-airway, bronchiolar, and alveolar injury with pulmonary edema can usually be differentiated on the basis of physical examination findings. Based on such findings, rescuers can determine the best initial approach to manage the victim's airway and respiratory distress.

Why is the patient's circulation depressed?   Emergency medical technicians and paramedics often care for patients with depressed circulation and other life-threatening conditions. Following trauma, depressed circulation and hypoperfusion are usually due to blood loss and hypovolemia. In severely ill medical patients, the causes of tissue hypoperfusion are more likely to include dehydration, pump failure resulting from primary heart disease, or loss of vascular tone.

Circulatory disturbances can also result from hazardous materials exposures. Violent trauma with blood loss can accompany chemicals accidents. Toxic skin burns, like thermal burns, lead to fluid loss and dehydration. Compromise of the heart's function can occur from the toxic effects of chemicals (such as arsenic) that act directly on the heart muscle. Other chemicals cause disturbed heart rhythms. In victims with underlying coronary artery disease, the stress of chemical exposure can cause myocardial infarction and congestive heart failure. Chemicals that act as anesthetics alter the nervous system's control of vascular tone and lead to vascular collapse.

It is not always possible to determine the specific reason for circulatory compromise in every patient. Observations made during the assessment, however, can suggest likely causes. Such observations can also suggest approaches for victim management.

Has the patient suffered trauma?   It is easy to ignore the possibility of trauma in toxic exposure victims because toxic emergencies are relatively uncommon. Some have a tendency to view these emergencies as special events that are unrelated to commoner emergency situations. As a result, rescuers may fail to approach victims in standard and orderly ways. In addition, rescuers sometimes do not look for multiple causes of a patient's distress. They may prefer to think that victims suffer only a single, important injury.

Trauma and hazardous material exposures can often occur together, however. More than half of all hazardous materials accidents occur during transportation. Hence, every vehicular accident poses the risk of also being a hazardous materials incident. Victims of such vehicular accidents can suffer both trauma and toxic exposure. In a similar way, victims of fires, explosions, and industrial accidents at chemical plants and storage facilities can suffer both toxic exposure and trauma.

It is important that EMS responders promptly recognize the presence of trauma in exposure victims and the presence of exposure injury in trauma victims. Failure to recognize and respond to both types of injury can compromise a victim's survival.

Components of the secondary survey for hazardous materials victims.   A complete secondary survey should be carried out in all victims. Rescuers wearing fully encapsulating entry suits and other personal protective equipment, however, are unable to perform most of the survey. Therefore, it is often necessary to delay the secondary survey of a hazardous materials exposure victim until decontamination has been completed.

The secondary survey can be helpful in evaluating hazardous materials victims. Some specific survey components help to characterize the type of exposure and the severity of injuries that resulted. Survey components that are particularly useful are described subsequently. Components of the secondary survey are illustrated in Figure 10–1.

Examination of the *head* may reveal evidence of trauma. For example, skull fractures that cause depressions or deformities of the skull bone can be easily palpated. Blood or clear cerebral spinal fluid visualized in the ear canals or nose also suggest head trauma with fracture. Likewise, head trauma with intracranial bleeding is likely in patients with abnormal findings such as racoon's eyes (ecchymoses or bruises around the eye orbits) or Battle's sign (ecchymoses or

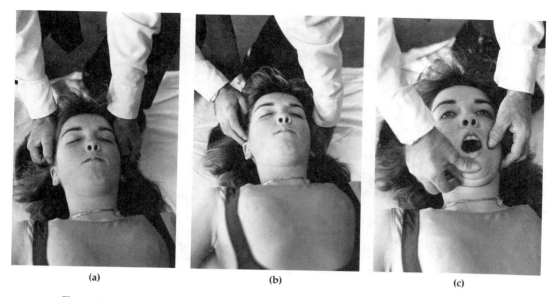

Figure 10–1 Examination of head. (a) Check for fractures and bleeding; examine ears. (b) Palpate neck. (c) Examine mouth for loose or broken teeth; check airway.

bruises behind the ears). Examination of the *eyes* may reveal unequal pupils, suggesting the presence of head injury or stroke. Dilated, unresponsive pupils are commonly associated with lack of oxygen and cerebral anoxia. Exposure to vesicant gases and tear gases lead to intense lacrimation, pain, and blurred vision. Acids and alkali splashed into the eye can cause opacification of the cornea. Altered vision and delayed blindness can result from methanol exposure.

COMPONENTS OF THE SECONDARY SURVEY

1. Examination of head
2. Examination of eyes
3. Examination of skin
4. Examination of thorax
5. Examination of lungs
6. Examination of abdomen
7. Examination of nervous system
8. Examination of pelvis and extremities

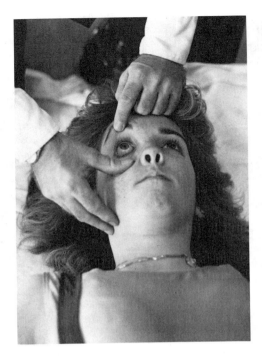

Figure 10–1.2 Examination of eyes. Pupils are checked for equality and reaction to light. Check for racoon's eyes and opacification.

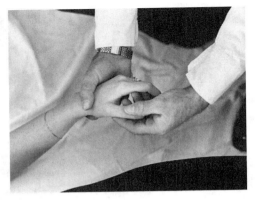

Figure 10–1.3 Examination of skin. Check for cyanosis, staining, sloughing, burns, pallor, flushing, blisters, and fissures.

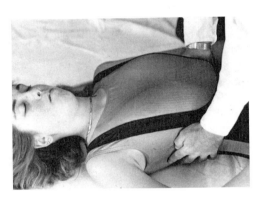

Figure 10–1.4 Examination of thorax. Compress chest to locate any rib fractures. Listen to chest for abnormalities of the heart, lungs, and airways.

Because the skin is often directly affected by hazardous chemicals, examination of the *skin* is a crucial component of the secondary survey. Skin abnormalities that can result from exposure to hazardous materials include staining, blisters, sloughing, burns, and fissures. The skin can also reveal the effects of chemicals that have affected organs other than the skin. For example, cyanosis, pallor, and flushing are common skin findings that result from many types of toxic exposure.

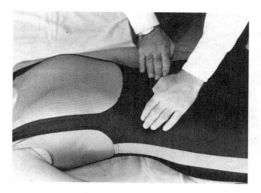

Figure 10–1.5 Examination of abdomen. Palpate abdomen for signs of penetration, pain, and abnormalities.

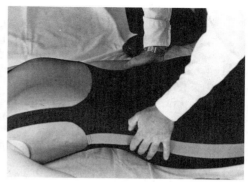

Figure 10–1.6 Examination of pelvis. Palpate pelvis for signs of fracture.

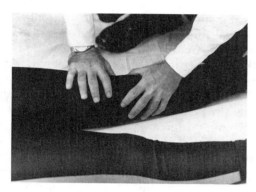

Figure 10–1.7 Examination of extremities. Palpate arms and legs for signs of bleeding, fractures, and pain.

Cyanosis can result from chemical effects on the lungs or the blood cells and hemoglobin. Exposure to nitrites, nitrates, and other nitrogen-containing compounds can cause cyanosis. Rescuers should examine the lips, mucous membranes, and fingernail beds for the presence of cyanosis. Cyanotic patients without signs of dyspnea or respiratory insufficiency should be suspected of having suffered toxic exposure.

Examination of the *thorax* can reveal traumatic injuries. Abnormalities of the heart, lungs, and airways can also be found. All patients should undergo a thorough chest examination. Chest wall deformities and crepitation are clues to underlying trauma. Asymmetrically decreased breath sounds suggest pneumo-thorax, a possible complication of both blunt and sharp trauma. Distant heart sounds associated with hypotension and distended neck veins suggest trau-matic pneumomediastinum or cardiac tamponade.

The heart rhythm may be altered by toxic exposures. For example, solvents such as toluene and benzene sensitize the heart to epinephrine and cause devel-opment of rapid dysrhythmia including ventricular fibrillation. Insecticides, con-versely, produce bradycardia leading to hypotension and shock. Chemicals that limit the blood's ability to carry oxygen (such as carbon monoxide) can lead to cardiac ischemia, myocardial infarction, and heart failure.

Pulmonary edema can result from either primary heart disease or chemical injury to the lungs. Unfortunately, it is not possible to separate these two forms of pulmonary edema on the basis of a clinical examination. When possible, car-diac monitoring should be an important part of the care provided to exposure victims.

Examination of the *lungs* is an essential part of the secondary survey. As described in chapter 15, hazardous materials exposure can lead to a wide range of respiratory injuries. Several abnormalities can be revealed by auscultation of the lungs. For example, some chemical inhalations cause bronchiolar damage and asthmalike symptoms. In these cases, examination findings include wheez-ing and delayed exhalation. In other cases, the presence of pulmonary edema may be suspected because crackles (or rales) are heard in the lungs.

Some of the pulmonary effects of chemical inhalations, especially pulmo-nary edema, can be delayed in onset. In such cases, the secondary survey pro-vides an additional value by establishing a functional baseline for each victim. The meaning of later examinations is increased by the availability of that baseline to which later findings can be compared. That is helpful for detecting subtle changes and recognizing the development of delayed-onset pulmonary injuries.

Examination of the *abdomen* often reveals findings that are nonspecific and sometimes difficult to interpret. For example, many different types of chemicals cause nausea, vomiting, and diarrhea. Moreover, ingestion of many chemicals of various types cause intense upper-gastrointestinal effects and bleeding. Ac-cordingly, such complaints and findings are usually so nonspecific that they are not very useful.

In other cases, however, exposure leads to characteristic and readily identi-fied sets of symptoms. For example, exposure to organophosphate and related insecticides causes profound diarrhea and sharp, crampy abdominal pain as well as increased amounts of urination, lacrimation, and salivation. Arsenic poi-soning, regardless of the exposure route, can cause intense abdominal com-plaints, profuse gastrointestinal bleeding, and cardiovascular collapse.

Many chemicals can cause liver abnormalities. In most cases, those effects are delayed for hours or days after exposure. In a few rare cases, such as expo-sure to arsine, tenderness over the liver and jaundice are early findings.

Assessment of abdominal complaints and abnormalities after toxic exposure usually requires repeat examinations and laboratory testing. Precise diagnosis is usually not possible without use of the facilities of a hospital.

Examination of the *nervous system* is of particular importance in victims who have suffered loss of consciousness, loss of motor control, disorientation, and other nervous system abnormalities. Soft neurological symptoms (such as dizziness, lightheadedness, or confusion) have been described after exposure to many hazardous chemicals of different types. Some effects are due to the direct action of chemicals on the central nervous system, as occurs with alcohol intoxication. In other cases, nervous system effects are due to electrolyte alterations (such as seizures caused by low blood calcium) or lack of oxygen. Victims can also suffer from hysterical symptoms and other effects of anxiety and fear resulting from the psychological impact of an incident that is viewed as life threatening.

The neurological component of the secondary survey is also important as a baseline against which later examinations of the patient can be compared. This is true for all patients with CNS disorders including more common conditions such as strokes and head trauma. In these patients, changing neurological signs and function have prognostic and diagnostic importance, and must be recognized.

Hazardous materials are unlikely to have acute toxic effects on the *pelvis or extremities*. Those structures, however, should be included during the secondary examination of victims. Of particular concern is the possibility of traumatic injuries. Fractures of the pelvis or femur, for example, can result in collections of large volumes of blood and edema fluid in the soft tissues. These fluid shifts, which can cause hypovolemia and shock, may go unrecognized unless a thorough examination is performed. Trauma can also result in neurovascular compromise of limbs that require urgent surgical repair and must be promptly recognized by rescuers.

CLINICAL IMPRESSION

The findings from the subjective interview and objective examination are brought together to formulate a clinical impression of the patient's condition. In some cases of hazardous materials exposure, it is possible for rescuers to formulate a specific impression. For example, enough information may be available to conclude that a patient has suffered corrosive burns of the eyes. In other cases, it may be uncertain whether the patient actually suffered any form of toxic exposure. For example, an unconscious victim with signs of pulmonary edema may have suffered inhalation injury, heart failure, or both.

When too little information is available to formulate a specific clinical impression, rescuers should at least summarize their actual findings. A clear statement should be made of the reasons that exposure injury has been suspected. It is tempting to conclude that a victim found in a contaminated place has suffered toxic exposure, but that is not always the case. Rescuers should consider the possibility that trauma, rather than toxic exposure, is the cause of a victim's condition.

The clinical impression should be developed carefully and thoughtfully. It will become the basis for choosing patient management strategies. Accordingly, if that impression is not well developed or ignores important alternative diagnostic possibilities, then victims are unlikely to receive proper and necessary care.

TREATMENT PLAN

The final phase of patient assessment involves the development of an appropriate and regionally accepted emergency treatment plan. The goals of the plan should be to maintain adequate oxygenation of tissues, control blood loss, improve circulation, and, when appropriate, reverse toxic effects. A proper plan guides the management and care of victims until they can be transported to definitive medical care facilities such as a local hospital emergency department.

The plan must be appropriate to the skill levels of the emergency responders providing care to the victim. It should at least address those skills and techniques needed to control the victim's airway, assure adequate patient ventilation, and stop bleeding. The ability to reverse shock by means of intravenous infusions or compression garments is also desirable. In a few cases, the administration of antidotal medications can be life saving. Proper application of these techniques will result in the stabilization of patients for enough time to permit definitive care to be provided.

SUMMARY

A systematic approach to patient assessment will enable the emergency responder to recognize the victim's present condition and potential for improvement, take appropriate steps for stabilization at the scene, and favorably impact the long-range outcome. It is important that rescuers consider hazardous materials exposure as a cause of illness in all victims, and that more conventional illnesses and trauma also be considered in victims of toxic exposure.

The variety, complexity, and volume of hazardous materials in our world create a potential for toxic injury or illness at any emergency. A general knowledge of the effects of chemicals, an awareness of their potential for harm, and proficiency in the basic emergency response techniques will greatly enhance a rescuer's efforts to provide proper care.

REFERENCES

Advanced Trauma Life Support Student Manual. Chicago, Ill.: American College of Surgeons, 1988.

BRONSTEIN, ALVIN C., and PHILLIP L. CURRANCE, *Emergency Care for Hazardous Materials Exposure.* St. Louis: The C. V. Mosby Company, 1988.

CARLSON, GENE P., ed., *HazMat Response Team Leak and Spill Guide:* Stillwater, Okla: Fire Protection Publications, 1984.

DONE, ALAN K., "Solving the Poison Puzzle," *Emerg. Med.,* February 1979, 305–314.

GRANT, HARVEY D., RUBERT H. MURRAY, and J. DAVID BERGERON, *Emergency Care.* Englewood Cliffs, N.J.: Prentice-Hall, Inc. 1986.

NOLL, GREGORY G., MICHAEL S. HILDEBRAND, and James G. Yvorra, *Hazardous Materials: Managing the Incident.* Stillwater, Okla: Fire Protection Publications, 1988.

PHILLIPS, CHARLES, *Basic Life Support Skills Manual.* Englewood Cliffs, N.J.: Prentice Hall, Inc., 1986.

Proceedings of "The Medical Management of HazMat Incidents," presented by Michael S. Hildebrand, American Petroleum Institute, and Prince George Fire Department's Hazardous Materials Response Team; sponsored by the EMS degree program, George Washington University, Washington, D.C., June 1988.

PROCEDURES

FOR RAPID EXTRICATION

CHAPTER 11

GOAL: On completion of this chapter the student will understand those aspects of incident assessment and patient assessment that are necessary to decide whether rapid extrication should be performed. The student will also be able to perform an extrication procedure.

OBJECTIVES:

Specifically, the student will be able to

- Discuss the necessary information that rescuers must obtain to plan a rescue and make extrication decisions
- Name the situations in which rapid extrication should be considered
- Describe one set of techniques for axial stabilization and skeletal immobilization using a long spine board
- Describe a technique for stabilization and immobilization using a scoop-type stretcher
- Describe the techniques for rapid extrication from a vehicle

OVERVIEW

This chapter is concerned with the role of rapid extrication in the management of hazardous materials exposure victims. We first discuss aspects of incident and victim assessment that help determine whether victims require rapid extrication. Then we review immobilization and rapid extrication techniques.

    Rapid extrication is a method for moving victims as quickly as possible from an incident site without causing additional harm. It is a critically important step in the management of trauma patients. It is also important in the care of hazardous materials victims.

Emergency response plans often require removal of exposure victims from contaminated places without first immobilizing them. Such response plans ignore the possibility that chemical victims may need specific trauma management and protection from further injury. The combination of exposure and trauma injury is a common occurrence.

Whenever possible, victims of trauma and victims of hazardous materials exposure who are suspected of trauma should have rapid assessment and proper immobilization before being moved.

RAPID ASSESSMENT

Some victims suffer both chemical exposure and trauma as a result of violent industrial accidents. For example, both injury types can be caused by explosions, fires, and other accidents at industrial plants. Likewise, both can result from transportation accidents such as freight train derailments and vehicular collisions involving chemical tank trucks. Chemical spills and exposures resulting from transportation accidents are common. In recent years, these accidents have represented more than half of all reported hazardous materials incidents.

In such situations, it is important that neither the trauma nor the chemical exposure be ignored because of their simultaneous presence. In the patient assessment and survey, it is essential that rescuers consider the possible presence of both toxic exposure and trauma.

During rapid assessment, rescuers should identify situations requiring rapid extrication. The decision to perform rapid extrication of hazardous materials victims is based on the three following considerations:

- Condition of patient
- Nature of hazardous material
- Safety of environment

Information needed to plan the rescue and make extrication decisions should routinely be obtained during incident assessment (see chapter 9). That information should include the following:

- Identification of the chemical involved in the incident
- Determination of the duration of exposure and likely exposure concentration levels
- Toxicity, health risks of the chemical, and the need for and availability of specific antidotes

- Environmental concerns such as air concentration of the chemical at the accident scene and the likely dispersion of the chemical
- Clinical condition of the patient (especially the vital signs), and when appropriate, trauma score or equivalent field triage assessment

Obtaining this information is critical to the rescue. With adequate information, rescuers can decide whether it is possible to enter the contaminated place safely to care for victims. Rescuers should only enter contaminated places when they have appropriate personal protective equipment available. The rescuers must also know how to use that protective equipment. Once rescuers have established that they can safely enter a contaminated zone, then they must decide whether victims can be managed safely at the incident scene or must first be extricated.

Rapid extrication should be considered for exposure victims in critically unstable clinical conditions, whether resulting from hazardous materials intoxication or trauma. Such unstable and critical conditions are usually identified during the primary survey. Assessment of all victims must begin with evaluation of airway, breathing, circulation, and disability such as level of consciousness. Examples of such conditions are presented subsequently:

1. Acute respiratory distress, as indicated by a respiratory rate of greater than 29 or less than 8 breaths per minute, is an indication for rapid extrication.

2. Rapid extrication should be considered for victims suffering hypotension and compromised circulation, as indicated by a systolic blood pressure below 80 mm Hg, the absence of palpable pulses, or the presence of other abnormalities that suggest inadequate tissue perfusion. Such abnormalities may include altered level of consciousness, abnormal skin color, and weak arterial pulses.

   - Severe hypotension and hypovolemia impair cerebral perfusion and cause dulled thinking and unconsciousness. A conscious patient who thinks clearly has at least adequate perfusion to maintain brain functions.
   - The presence of pink skin is a sign of adequate tissue perfusion. Severely hypovolemic and hypotensive patients have ashen, gray skin and pale, blood-drained extremities.
   - A full, slow, regular pulse in a peripheral artery usually indicates adequate blood volume and cardiac output. By contrast, a rapid and thready pulse is often a sign of hypovolemia or hypotension. Presence of a radial pulse was thought to indicate a systolic blood pressure greater than 80 to 90 mm Hg, but this has not been verified.

3. Rapid extrication and transport may be required by potentially lethal exposures, such as that resulting from hydrogen cyanide, for which specific antidotal treatments are necessary but not available at the incident site.

4. Rapid extrication should also be considered for exposure victims who have

been trapped in an environment that poses a lethal risk to them. Examples of such situations follow.

- Victims exposed to high air concentrations of hazardous chemicals are at risk of rapid death. In particular, victims exposed to concentrations exceeding the IDLH level or the STEL level are candidates for rapid extrication.
- Victims exposed to potentially explosive or flammable air concentrations of hazardous chemicals, especially when the environmental temperatures approximate or exceed the chemicals' autoignition temperature, are at great danger and should be rapidly extricated if possible.

RAPID EXTRICATION

Unnecessary body movement can worsen the clinical condition of traumatized individuals. Trauma victims with spinal injuries can suffer irreparable harm to the spinal cord following twisting or flexion of the spine. In long bone fractures, particularly open fractures, unprotected movement of the fractured part can cause limb-threatening vascular and neurological injury.

To assure that injury is not caused or worsened by rescuers moving trauma patients, axial stabilization and skeletal immobilization should be performed. Chemical exposure victims suspected of having suffered trauma should receive the same care. This is particularly true in situations that do not permit a complete assessment and survey before transporting the patient.

The following describes one set of techniques for axial stabilization and skeletal immobilization using a long spine board. Because a long board is found on almost every ambulance, EMS personnel should be familiar with its use. Evidence discussed subsequently, however, suggests that scoop-type stretchers are preferable to long boards for spinal injury victims. EMS personnel should also know how to use scoop stretchers.

1. Straighten the neck to the neutral position. **If resistance is felt, stop!** Splint the neck in that position (Figure 11–1a).
2. Apply cervical collar and head immobilizer in conjunction with a long board or scoop-style stretcher.
3. Fractures are splinted by immobilizing the joint above and the joint below the fracture site. Placing the victim on a long board results in the body being splinted from head to toe.
4. Victims should be placed on a long board in the supine position. This enables the emergency responder to assess the victim's level of consciousness and respiratory rate more easily. The supine position also allows for greater depth of respiration without resistance. Occasional exceptions to the supine position rule exist such as a victim with an object impaled in his or her back; emergency responders should *not* remove impaled objects.

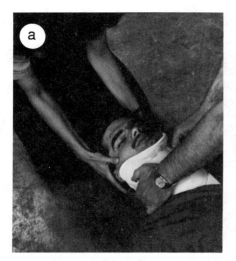

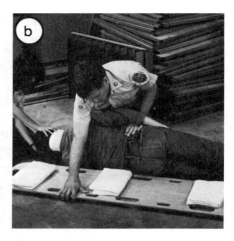

Figure 11–1 (a) First emergency medical technician (EMT) maintains an open airway and manual traction while second EMT applies an extrication collar. (b) The patient is rolled toward second emergency medical technician, and the long spine board is placed as far under the patient as possible. (c) Once the patient has been positioned, he or she should be secured to the board.

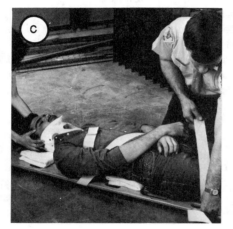

5. The following describes a commonly practiced method for log rolling a patient onto a long spine board. Evidence discussed later indicates that log rolling poses risk of injury to spinal trauma victims. Therefore, immobilization devices such as scoop stretchers that do not require log rolling are preferred over long spine boards.

   • Place the board alongside the victim so that the distal end of the board is adjacent to the victim's knees.
   • One rescuer maintains head stabilization, and the other rescuer log rolls the victim. The victim is rolled toward the second rescuer. The arm on the side to which the victim is rolled should be left alongside the body. Do not elevate the arm over the head. Doing so puts tension

on the muscles that attach to the spinal processes and can cause the vertebral column to be pulled laterally.

- Place the board as far under the patient as possible (Figure 11–1b).
- Roll the patient on to the board in a supine position. At this stage of the process, the patient's head should be below the top of the board. The patient's body should not yet lie on the middle of the board.
- While the first rescuer continues to hold the head in the neutral position, the second rescuer slides the patient up the board. The patient should be moved diagonally, 6 to 8 inches at a time. Each successive slide should be angled so that the patient moves toward the board's center.
- Once positioned, the patient should be secured to the board (Figure 11–1c).

6. The victim can now be moved rapidly to a safer site where full assessment can be carried out and treatment can begin.

A problem with the use of long spine boards is the need to log roll victims onto the board. It is difficult for two emergency medical technicians to position a victim on a long board properly without using that rolling procedure. Although supposedly safe, log rolling can cause movement and displacement of the spine. Even when performed by a team of four experienced EMS personnel, log rolling caused enough movement in unstable spine fractures to cause neurological damage.

By contrast, the scoop-type stretcher can be used by two emergency medical technicians without requiring log rolls or other movements of the victim's body. The following describes a technique for stabilization and immobilization using a scoop-type stretcher:

1. Straighten the neck to the neutral position. **If resistance is felt, stop!** Splint the neck in that position.

2. Apply cervical collar and head immobilizer in conjunction with a scoop-style stretcher.

3. Fractures are splinted by immobilizing the joint above and the joint below the fracture site. Placing the victim on a scoop-style stretcher results in the body being splinted from head to toe.

4. Victims should be placed as straight as possible in the supine position. The arms should be secured in place.

5. The stretcher's length should be adjusted to fit the patient. Then the stretcher's two halves are separated and slid underneath the patient. The two halves are then latched together beginning at the head and moving down toward the feet. The head support should be adjusted and the patient is then strapped to the stretcher (Figure 11–2,a–d).

6. The victim can now be moved rapidly to a safer site where full assessment can be carried out and treatment can begin.

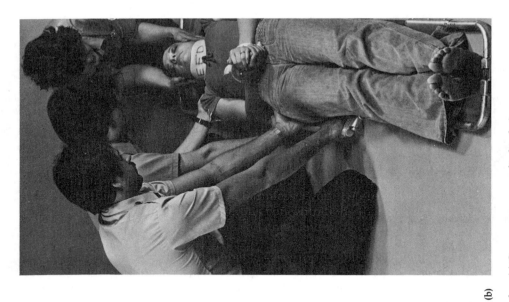

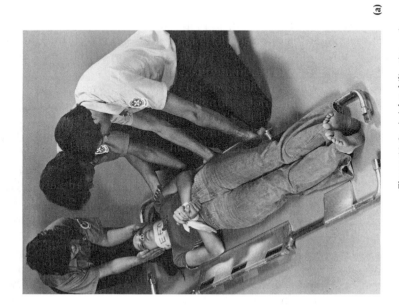

(a)

(b)

Figure 11-2 Axial stabilization using scoop stretcher. (a) One emergency medical technician carefully supports the patient's head while half of the stretcher is positioned. (b) The second half of the stretcher is locked into the first.

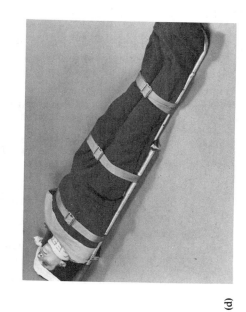

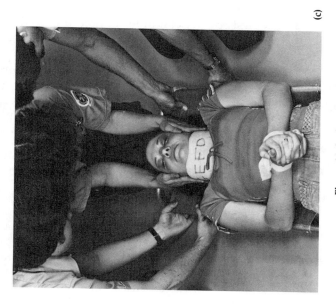

(c)

(d)

Figure 11-2 (*continued*) (c) The vinyl head support is properly positioned. (d) The patient properly positioned, covered, and secured on a scoop-style stretcher.

RAPID VEHICULAR EXTRICATION

More than half of all hazardous materials accidents occur during transportation. The combination of vehicular trauma and hazardous materials exposure can readily occur. Rapid extrication of a victim from a vehicle poses a somewhat more difficult challenge to rescuers. The following describes a technique for three emergency medical technicians to perform rapid vehicular extrication. The steps are illustrated in Figure 11–3,a–f.

1. The first rescuer should accomplish axial stabilization of the head and neck from outside the vehicle.
2. The second rescuer applies a cervical collar.
3. While the first rescuer continues to hold the head and neck, the second rescuer prepares to rotate the victim. That rescuer places one hand between the victim's back and the vehicle seat, and reaches across and behind to the victim's far hip. The rescuer's other hand is placed on the victim's chest to help stabilize the body.
4. The third rescuer enters the vehicle's passenger compartment on the side opposite the second rescuer. He or she holds the victim's legs and prepares to help rotate the victim.
5. With the rescuer at the head in charge, the victim is rotated a few degrees at a time until the back can be lowered unobstructed to a long board.
6. The first rescuer continues to hold the head while the victim is being lowered. Once the victim is supine and placed on the long board, the head will be supported in the neutral position.
7. The second rescuer supports the victim's upper body as it is lowered to the board.
8. While the first rescuer maintains head stabilization, the second rescuer applies pressure to the pelvic girdle and slides the patient up the board a few inches at a time. The patient will be moved until his or her head is at the top of the board.

SUMMARY

Trauma and hazardous materials exposure can occur together. Rescuers should suspect trauma in all severe exposure victims. Because exposure to hazardous materials may require rapid removal of victims from contaminated places, rescuers at hazardous materials incidents should be prepared to perform rapid extrication. The need for rapid extrication is determined by the information obtained by rescuers during incident assessment. The same information should be used to decide whether rescuers can safely enter a contaminated area.

Several techniques are available for axial stabilization and skeletal immobi-

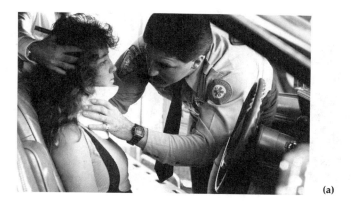

(a)

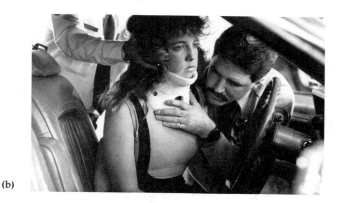

(b)

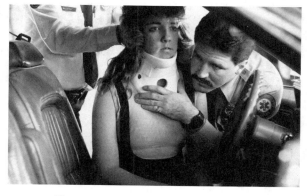

(c)

Figure 11–3 Rapid vehicular extrication. (a) Axial stabilization of the head and neck. (b) Second rescuer places right hand between patient's back and vehicle seat, reaching around to the patient's right hip. The left hand is placed on the patient's chest for stabilization. (c) With rescuer at head maintaining stabilization, the patient is turned toward the inside of the vehicle a few degrees at a time.

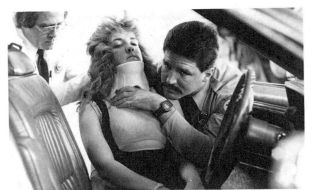

(d)

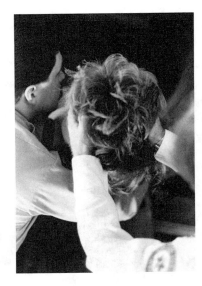

(e)

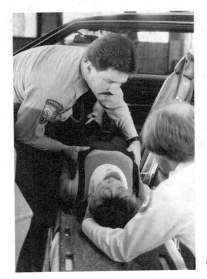

(f)

Figure 11–3 Rapid vehicular extrication (*continued*). (d) The rescuer at the head continues to support the head while the patient is being lowered. (e) The patient is turned completely toward the inside of the vehicle. (f) Second rescuer grabs the pelvic girdle and slides the patient up the board a few inches at a time.

lization. The commonest one involves a long spine board. This equipment often requires log rolling the victim. Because log rolling can lead to spinal injuries, techniques that do not require log rolling, such as use of a scoop-type stretcher, are preferred.

REFERENCES

Advanced Trauma Life Support Student Manual. Chicago: American College of Surgeons, 1988.

BRONSTEIN, ALVIN C., and PHILLIP L. CURRANCE, *Emergency Care for Hazardous Materials Exposure.* St. Louis: The C. V. Mosby Company, 1988.

CARLSON, GENE P., ed., *HazMat Response Team Leak and Spill Guide.* Stillwater, Okla.: Fire Protection Publications, 1984.

GRANT, HARVEY D., ROBERT H. MURRAY, and J. DAVID BERGERON, *Emergency Care.* Englewood Cliffs, N.J.: Prentice Hall, Inc., 1986.

McGUIRE, ROBERT A., SHIRLEY NEVILLE, BARTH A. GREEN, and CLARK WATTS, ''Spinal instability and the log-rolling technique'' *Rescue-EMS News,* (1988) no 14.

NOLL, GREGORY G., MICHAEL S. HILDEBRAND, and JAMES G. YVORRA, *Hazardous Materials: Managing the Incident.* Stillwater, Okla.: Fire Protection Publications, 1988.

PHILLIPS, CHARLES, *Basic Life Support: Skills Manual.* Englewood Cliffs, N.J.: Prentice Hall, Inc., 1986.

Proceedings of ''The Medical Management of HazMat Incidents,'' presented by Michael S. Hildebrand, American Petroleum Institute, and Prince George Fire Department's Hazardous Materials Response Team; sponsored by the EMS degree program, George Washington University, Washington, D.C., June 1988.

PROCEDURES FOR DECONTAMINATION

GOAL: On completion of this chapter the student will be able to define decontamination, discuss the significance of decontamination, and describe basic decontamination procedures.

OBJECTIVES:

Specifically, the student will be able to

- Discuss the importance of a preincident plan
- Describe the issues to be addressed in an incident plan
- Describe a typical equipment list for a large-scale decontamination procedure
- Name some environmental concerns that may impact on the ways in which decontamination is performed
- Name the methods by which decontamination can be accomplished and the appropriateness of each
- Describe the basic procedures for moving rescuers, victims, tools, and equipment along the decontamination route
- Name agencies that should be involved in the cleanup procedures
- Discuss debriefing and the importance of medical surveillance of rescuers

OVERVIEW

This chapter considers the role and implementation of decontamination efforts at hazardous materials incidents. First, some preincident planning issues that can contribute to successful decontamination efforts are considered. Then, some operational issues are discussed that are relevant to setting up and carrying out decontamination. Finally, one "model" for a large-scale decontamination is presented.

Decontamination is essential for successfully managing a hazardous materials incident. The scope and methods of the necessary decontamination effort will be determined for each situation by the specific chemicals involved, the nature of the releases, and the number of people affected.

In some situations, decontamination may be accomplished by having the victim wash under a shower. That, for example, might be appropriate management for a single worker sprayed by an acid or alkali. Conversely, a complex system of restricted access areas and a stepwise decontamination procedure may be required when large numbers of people and equipment have been exposed to a highly reactive and lethal compound. In that case, it may also be necessary to contain the chemical so that environmental contamination is avoided.

Every hazardous materials incident, regardless of its size and nature, poses a probable need for decontamination. To assure that every incident receives appropriate decontamination, a standard approach should be used by rescuers. Decontamination can benefit greatly from preplanning and the use of standard operating procedures.

DECONTAMINATION

Decontamination is the systematic removal of hazardous materials from exposure victims, rescue personnel, equipment, and the environment. Disposal of the hazards is also part of the decontamination process. Materials requiring decontamination can include the following:

1. Hazardous chemicals

2. Biologic hazards

3. Radiologic hazards

Thousands of *hazardous chemicals* exist that can cause injury to exposed persons. In most cases, severe injury or death occurs only when victims have been exposed to large amounts of chemicals for prolonged periods. In such cases, decontamination can remove the chemical before it has caused harm or before harm is severe.

A few lethal chemicals can cause death after even brief exposure to small quantities. Prompt decontamination in those situations may be life saving. In addition, decontamination and containment prevents their spread to rescuers and others.

Biologic hazards include bacteria, viruses, and materials that they produce. Many laboratories and research centers routinely experiment with organisms that cause infections and illness. New technologies in the biologic sciences (such as gene splitting) have allowed the production and storage of large quantities of active hormones and other biologic materials. Accidents involving biologic laboratories, production centers, or vehicles transporting these biologic hazards substances can result in important contamination.

We are all aware of the possibilities of accidents causing contamination by *radiologic hazards.* Recent nuclear accidents at the Three-Mile Island and Chernobyl power plants serve as reminders of the large-scale dangers of radiologic technology. Great potential for many smaller radiation accidents also exists—for example, those involving vehicles transporting nuclear materials and wastes on highways. Decontamination of victims involved in such radiation accidents can be important to restrict the spread of the radiation.

In general, recommended procedures for decontamination of exposure victims are the same for all three types of hazardous materials. Following radiation exposures, patients should be evaluated by a radiation physicist who should determine that decontamination has been adequate. Specialized medical assessments may be necessary to determine the need for further decontamination following exposure to biologic agents.

PLAN FOR DECONTAMINATION

A successful decontamination effort, especially for a large spill or toxic hazard, requires the cooperative effort of numerous emergency responders. Trained personnel must perform a wide range of tasks including identification of the hazardous material, assessment of its effects, and its actual removal and disposal. Adequate amounts of specialized equipment (such as chemical protective clothing, washing materials, and containment tanks) must be made rapidly available. All responders who may become contaminated must understand how and when to go through decontamination.

To carry out a large decontamination effort effectively, it is essential that a *preincident plan* be developed for each community and hazardous material site. The use of standard operating procedures permits rescue personnel to organize and manage hazardous materials incidents without confusion. Even for small accidents, such as those involving a single victim and little if any risk of environmental contamination, a systematic plan helps to assure that all needed decontamination steps are provided to victims. See Appendix 2 for a description of an incident command system.

Most communities have been required to perform such planning as part of the local emergency response plans mandated by the SARA. When such planning has been carried out, SARA's local emergency planning councils can identify the locations and types of hazardous materials in each community. Local emergency responders can then plan decontamination procedures for the chemicals with which they are most likely to deal. They can also identify the types, quantities, and location of equipment that would be needed for worst-case situations.

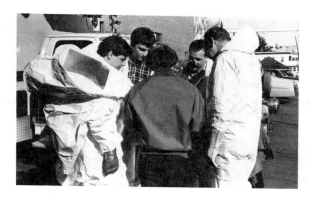

Figure 12–1 Before entering the contaminated area, rescuers meet to develop a rescue plan. This plan will address all facets of decontamination.

Preplanning the complex steps of decontamination helps responders to be ready to perform. It also increases the likelihood that necessary equipment and tools will be available. Figure 12–1 illustrates an emergency team designing a rescue plan.

TYPES OF DECONTAMINATION

Different methods exist by which decontamination can be accomplished. Five methods are described subsequently. The choice of the most appropriate method for a given situation depends on the specific nature of the hazardous materials involved. In some situations, only a single method is needed. In others, a combination of methods should be used. Techniques that are useful for removing contaminants from equipment may be hazardous to exposure victims.

1. *Mechanical removal:* Brushing off and wiping away visible contaminants are two fast and effective ways to begin decontamination. This is particularly useful for removing solid contaminants such as dusts and powders. It can also be used to remove liquids: Rapidly wiping spilt acid off the skin with a cloth decreases the severity of the burn caused by that acid.

This method poses the risk of depositing solid contaminants on the ground. It can also cause dusts to become airborne and spread to other areas and expose new victims.

2. *Dilution:* The most widely used form of decontamination is washing with water, which removes the contaminant while diluting it. Generally, dilution with water is the safest means to remove contaminants from a victim. Other solutions (such as saline and Ringer's lactate) serve as well, but the ready availability of water makes it the universal first choice.

A short list exists of chemicals for which water irrigation is not appropriate for decontamination. Water-reactive metals such as sodium and lithium produce heat and alkali that can cause thermal and chemical burns after contact with water. Victims exposed to these metals should not undergo water washing for decontamination.

Some chemicals are insoluble in water; therefore, water irrigation cannot effectively remove them from the skin of exposed individuals. In such cases, the addition of soap or mild detergent often makes an effective decontamination solution. In general, water-insoluble chemicals should be decontaminated using a soap or detergent wash.

In some cases, specific solvents are useful for decontaminating human victims. Rubbing alcohol, for example, can be used for water-insoluble contaminants; polyethylene glycol, a complex alcohol-like compound, is useful for removing corrosive compounds called phenols.

3. *Absorption:* This decontamination method is used for removing spilt chemicals from equipment and from the area around a spill. It has no role in the immediate management of exposure victims. Numerous absorbent materials, ranging from sand and soil to special manufactured compounds, are useful. Absorbents are generally inexpensive and readily available. They are especially effective for site cleanup because they prevent contaminants from spreading.

4. *Degradation:* It is possible to decontaminate a hazardous chemical by altering its chemical structure and converting it into a harmless compound or one that is more easily washed away. This technique is widely used for equipment decontamination but has little if any value for the management of exposure victims.

Neutralizing an acid by application of an alkali solution is an example of degradation. The acid and alkali combine and form a harmless salt. The chemical process of neutralization, however, yields enough heat to cause thermal burns. For that reason, neutralization should not be used for decontamination of victims with acid or alkali burns.

5. *Isolation and disposal:* Once a contaminating hazard has been contained, it must usually be removed from the site of the spill. Following absorption, for example, the absorbed contaminants should be carefully packaged and then removed to a disposal site. Likewise, the wash water used for chemical dilution should not be allowed to run off and carry chemicals into the soil or sewer system. Instead, that water should be collected for later disposal. This is critical to avoid spreading contamination beyond the spill site. Isolation and disposal play no direct role in decontaminating exposure victims.

PREPARATION FOR DECONTAMINATION

Preplanning, as described earlier, establishes a generally useful, systematic approach to decontamination. No two hazardous material incidents are exactly the same, however. The quantity and type of chemicals involved, the number of affected people, the terrain and surrounding environment, and even the time of day and weather serve to make each event unique. Therefore, almost every hazardous materials incident needs an incident plan that considers the specific emergency circumstances.

The incident plan should consider at least the following issues:

1. What are the hazards?

2. How large is the incident?

3. Are personnel and resources limited?

4. Does the environment require special protection?

Identification of the Hazards

The decontamination needs of a hazardous materials incident are largely determined by the materials involved. Identifying them, therefore, is of particular importance in formulating an incident plan. One rule of thumb is that chemicals should be researched in at least three separate sources of reference to be sure that all the health, reactivity, and flammability information has been obtained. Unfortunately, this is not always possible.

For large incidents, one or more emergency personnel should be devoted to identifying and researching the on-scene hazardous materials. Information about health risks and decontamination needs must be promptly transmitted to the decontamination team. It is important to know whether the chemical is water soluble, whether it can be absorbed from the skin, and whether it accumulates in the body or in the environment.

Evaluation of Incident Size

The size of the incident determines the scope of the decontamination efforts. When only a single victim and little likelihood that rescuers will become exposed to the chemical exist, then a simple decontamination setup (such as a shower stall) may be all that is needed.

Conversely, it may be necessary to decontaminate dozens of victims and still greater numbers of emergency responders. An explosion in a chemical factory, for example, might contaminate many workers and rescuers as well as great amounts of equipment. When estimating the number of persons who will need decontamination, remember that any rescuer who enters the contaminated area will require decontamination on the way outside.

As a general rule, it is better to decontaminate too many people than too few. The incident decontamination plan, however, must also be practical and efficient. It is almost never possible to decontaminate everyone at an incident.

Personnel and Resources

Emergency personnel must be assigned to supervise and carry out decontamination. Therefore, the size and scope of the decontamination setup is limited by the numbers of available personnel. The nine-station decontamination plan described later can only be used when enough personnel can properly staff each station. It is not always necessary to use all nine decontamination steps. The number of decontamination stations and the size of the decontamination team should be determined by the nature and size of the incident. In general, the number of responders assigned to the decontamination area must increase as the number involved at the incident increases.

Specific equipment needs also exist for decontamination. Showers must be available or constructed, run-off must be collected for disposal, and adequate amounts of equipment of various types must be ready at the site. The incident plan must consider the actual resources available. A typical equipment list for large-scale decontamination is presented.

1. Perimeter and sector markers

2. Absorbent

3. Water supply manifolds and delivery systems

4. Brushes

5. Soaps, detergents, and decontamination solutions

6. Disposal barrels

7. Run-off barriers

8. Plastic sheets and tarps

9. Containment pits

10. Communications equipment

11. Spinal immobilization boards

12. EMS and medical equipment

13. Lights

Special Environmental Concerns

Several types of environmental concerns may directly influence the ways in which decontamination is performed at an incident. Some of those concerns involve protecting the environment from chemical contamination. Others are focused on protecting victims and rescuers from the environment.

Selection of the decontamination site is one concern. It should be located upwind from the area of contamination. If this is not done and the site is mistakenly placed downwind from the contaminated area, then the decontamination area can become contaminated by wind-blown chemicals. When possible, the site should be located at a higher elevation than the contaminated zone. In that way, uncontained washing solution run-off will flow back toward the area of contamination and not into clean areas.

Some incidents will pose a risk to sources of drinking water (such as reservoirs or wells) and open running water (such as lakes and rivers). The decontamination site should be located as far as possible from such water supplies.

Environmental conditions can also pose risks to victims and rescuers. During freezing weather, for example, it may not be safe to perform out-of-doors washing of contaminated persons. It may be necessary to plan decontamination at an off-site location or inside a renovated vehicle such as a school bus. In such a case, part of the incident decontamination plan must include methods for transporting victims to the decontamination site and subsequent decontamination of the transport vehicles.

PERFORMANCE OF DECONTAMINATION

Decontamination is carried out in a series of steps or stations that begin at gross decontamination and end at the EMS treatment area (Figure 12–2). Each station employs its own decontamination personnel. The level of contamination at each should be less than at the previous station. Personnel should not move back and forth from higher to lower contamination areas without passing through decontamination. This guideline helps to prevent contamination of the decontamination stations. Decontamination personnel must pass through the decontamination process to exit the decontamination area.

Victims are transported from the hot zone to gross decontamination by members of the entry team. As victims move along the decontamination process, they are passed from one team of decontamination workers to another team at each decontamination station. Rarely, victims who have suffered severe trauma or poisoning must undergo rapid decontamination to permit rapid transport to a hospital. Even in those cases, however, the victims should be passed sequentially through all decontamination stations. Failure to do so risks contaminating the entire health care system as described later in chapter 14.

Presented subsequently is a nine-station decontamination sector plan that is typical of decontamination procedures that have been used at mass casualty chemical accidents. At a large incident, each station might be physically separate. At smaller ones, several of the stations may be combined. Generally, there should be at least two stations to the decontamination process.

Regardless of the number of decontamination stations, each decontamination step should be performed. This is so even when only a single exposure victim exists. One exception to this rule occurs when victims also suffer a life-threatening condition for which immediate medical attention is required. In that

9-Station Decontamination Procedure

STEPS

STATION 1. Rescuers enter decon area and mechanically remove contaminants from victims. Tools are dropped in tool drop area. Rescuers are in SCBA and protective clothing. **Proceed to Station 2.**

STATION 2. Gross Decontamination: Victims and rescue personnel are showered and/or scrubbed by decon personnel. Dilution is conducted inside diked area. Victims may be transported directly to Station 6. **Proceed to Station 3.**

STATION 3. Protective Clothing Removal: Rescuers remove protective clothing, clothing is isolated and labeled for later disposal. Clothing is placed on contaminated side. **Proceed to Station 4.**

STATION 4. SCBA Removal: Rescue personnel remove and isolate their SCBA. If re-entry is necessary, personnel don new SCBA from non-contaminated side. **Proceed to Station 5.**

STATION 5. Personnel Clothing Removal: All clothing and personal items are removed. Victims who have not been undressed are undressed here. All clothing and personal items are isolated in plastic bags and labeled for later disposal. **Proceed to Station 6.**

STATION 6. Body Washing: Full body washing is performed using soft scrub brushes or sponges and soap or mild detergent. Cleaning tools are bagged for later disposal. **Proceed to Station 7.**

STATION 7. Dry Off: Towels and sheets are used to dry off. Rescuers and victims are dressed in clean clothes. Towels/sheets are bagged for later disposal. **Proceed to Station 8.**

STATION 8. Medical Assessment: Rapid patient assessment is conducted by rescuers. Necessary stabilization procedures are accomplished. **Proceed to Station 9.**

STATION 9. Transport: Transfer of patient to hospital for medical attention or to recovery areas for rest and observation.

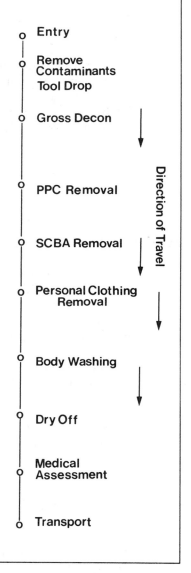

Figure 12–2 A graphic illustration of a nine-step decontamination procedure.

situation, victims can be transported to a definitive medical care facility after only gross decontamination. The EMS personnel, however, must be protected with appropriate personal protective equipment and the hospital must be prepared to treat a contaminated, critically ill patient. Following transport of the victim, the crew and ambulance must then undergo decontamination.

Station 1: Entry point and hot zone. A single entry point into the hot zone and a single exit leading to station 2 should exist. The entry team mechanically removes as much of the contaminants as possible from victims. Tools and equipment used in the hot zone are left in the tool drop area. Victims are then transported to station 2 for gross decontamination.

Station 2: Gross decontamination. Victims and rescue personnel should be showered or scrubbed by decontamination personnel wearing personal protective equipment. Washing is carried out primarily with water. Initially, victims should be washed while fully dressed. Removal of victims' contaminated clothing may then be performed. It is critical that overspray be minimized and runoff be contained.

Victims can then be transported directly to station 6 for further body washing. Rescue personnel who exit the hot zone must first pass through stations 3 to 5.

Station 3: Protective clothing removal. All protective clothing is removed, isolated in plastic bags, and labeled for later disposal. Depending on the severity of the hazardous incident, personnel may have donned multiple levels of protective clothing. Protective clothing should be removed in stages (removal of outer clothing in one location and then removal of inner clothing at another).

Station 4: SCBA removal. In this station, rescue personnel can remove and isolate their SCBA. Changeover and replacement SCBA can be obtained if re-entry is necessary.

Station 5: Personal clothing removal. Rescue personnel entering this station should remove all clothing and personal items such as rings and watches. Victims who were not undressed at station 2 should be undressed here. All clothing and personal items should be packaged in plastic bags and labeled for later disposal.

Station 6: Body washing. Full body washing is performed at this station. Soft scrub brushes or sponges and soap or mild detergent should be used. Special attention should be given to hair, groin, skin folds, and nail beds. Copious water rinsing should also be performed.

Station 7: Dry off.   Towels and sheets are used to dry off the entire body. A clean change of clothes should also be supplied. Disposable coveralls or hospital gowns are inexpensive and can be made available for this station.

Station 8: Medical assessment.   At this station emergency responders conduct a rapid patient assessment. Vital signs should be taken and compared to baseline values. All open wounds should be cleansed and bandaged. A thorough respiratory and cardiac evaluation must be done. Any poison control recommendations should be followed at this time. Necessary stabilization procedures should be accomplished in this station. EMS personnel working in this station should be in direct contact with medical control, poison centers, product specialists, and other appropriate advisory services.

Station 9: Transport for definitive care.   This is a transfer station to facilitate the transport of patients to hospitals for medical attention, or to recovery areas for rest and observation.

CLEANUP

Because of time and expense, most hazardous materials and emergency response teams act in only an advisory capacity during cleanup. Other response organizations likely to be involved in the cleanup of most incidents include local water treatment and sewer departments, and pollution control agencies. They should be notified promptly of all hazardous leaks and spills; in turn, they should monitor contamination of local water supplies and sewer run-off. Product specialists with expertise in the containment and environmental control of specific chemicals can provide helpful assistance during the cleanup process. See Appendix 3 for descriptions of containment and confinement techniques.

DEBRIEFING PROCESS

The last step in the resolution of a hazardous material incident is debriefing. As soon as possible after the incident, all participating personnel should be informed about the chemicals involved and their long- and short-term health effects. Medical surveillance scheduling should be established for eligible personnel. See Appendix 4 for information about OSHA's medical surveillance requirements. In addition, this is the time to review all phases of the incident to identify successful and unsuccessful techniques and procedures. Difficulties experienced in performing decontamination should be noted, and any necessary revisions to the preplan and the standard operating procedures should be made.

SUMMARY

Decontamination is an essential part of hazardous materials incidents. It is possible to construct general rules that serve as standard operating procedures for developing a decontamination process. The specific chemicals involved, the number of persons needing decontamination, and the personnel and resources available determine the actual decontamination procedures to be followed.

REFERENCES

BRONSTEIN, ALVIN C., and PHILLIP L. CURRANCE, *Emergency Care for Hazardous Materials Exposure*, St. Louis: The C. V. Mosby Company, 1988.

CARLSON, GENE P., ed., *HazMat Response Team Leak and Spill Guide.* Stillwater, Okla.: Fire Protection Publications, 1984.

NOLL, GREGORY G., MICHAEL S. HILDEBRAND, and JAMES G. YVORRA, *Hazardous Materials: Managing the Incident.* Stillwater, Okla.: Fire Protection Publications, 1988.

Proceedings of ''The Medical Management of HazMat Incidents,'' presented by Michael S. Hildebrand, American Petroleum Institute, and Prince George Fire Department's Hazardous Materials Response Team; sponsored by the EMS degree program, George Washington University, Washington, D.C., June 1988.

STUTZ, DOUGLAS R., and STANLEY J. JANUSZ, *Hazardous Materials Injuries: A Handbook for Pre-Hospital Care.* Beltsville, Md.: Bradford Communications, 1988.

FIELD STABILIZATION AND PROCEDURES FOR HAZARDOUS MATERIALS VICTIMS

CHAPTER 13

GOAL: On completion of this chapter the student will have an understanding of many of the life-and-limb–threatening health conditions caused by hazardous materials and will be able to describe appropriate EMS procedures for correcting those conditions.

OBJECTIVES:

Specifically, the student will be able to

- List three ways that hazardous materials can cause airway obstruction and the appropriate procedures used to correct obstruction when it occurs
- Describe two situations in which mouth-to-mouth rescue breathing can cause injury to a rescuer at a hazardous materials incident
- List five ways that hazardous materials exposure can cause hypotension and circulatory collapse
- Describe the proper method for performing irrigation of the eyes
- List three types of cardiac emergencies that can be caused by hazardous materials exposure
- List seven types of chemicals that can cause cardiac emergencies in hazardous materials victims
- Describe four antidotes for hazardous materials victims that could be used in an EMS system

OVERVIEW

This chapter describes some EMS procedures that are useful for the management of hazardous materials victims. First, management of a victim's airway, breathing, and circulation are discussed. Next, emergency procedures for the care of exposed skin and eye are considered. Then, emergency cardiac care issues and cardiac procedures are outlined. Finally, four antidotes of value in the prehospital care of exposure victims are presented.

The prehospital stabilization and management of hazardous materials victims should be based on knowledge and performance of standard EMS procedures and practice. As with other emergency patients, initial concerns must be directed to the "ABCs" of resuscitation: an open airway must be maintained with adequate breathing and circulation. After the ABCs have received attention, it is then appropriate for rescuers to consider other effects that hazardous materials may cause.

AIRWAY MANAGEMENT

Victims of hazardous materials exposure can suffer potentially life-threatening obstruction of the airway. It can result from several different pathological mechanisms such as the following:

1. Loss of consciousness

2. Direct injury to the upper airway

3. Excessive secretions

Appropriate emergency management of a victim's airway will depend on the type of injury that has been suffered.

Loss of Consciousness

Many chemicals can cause exposure victims to suffer CNS depression that results in loss of consciousness. As described in chapter 18, most of these chemicals are fat-soluble solvents. Others are enzyme poisons such as cyanide and hydrogen sulfide. In these patients, relaxation of the pharyngeal muscles permits the tongue to slide or fall backward into the pharynx, which can result in airway obstruction.

All unconscious victims are in danger of airway obstruction. For such victims, use of an oropharyngeal or nasopharyngeal airway is usually appropriate. An oropharyngeal airway should be used only for victims lacking an intact gag reflex. If that reflex is present, use of an oropharyngeal airway is likely to stimulate gagging and vomiting. Aspiration of vomitus into the lungs and severe lung injury can result. By contrast, a nasopharyngeal airway can often be used effectively and safely in patients with intact gag reflexes.

Victims must be closely monitored once an oropharyngeal airway has been inserted. Some solvents, such as toluene, can cause brief periods of unconsciousness or fluctuating levels of consciousness with relapsing episodes of coma. As consciousness returns, the danger increases that an inserted airway will cause gagging and aspiration. If evidence exists of gagging or vomiting, the airway must be immediately removed. When using an oropharyngeal airway, suction equipment should be immediately available to assure a rapid response if vomiting occurs.

In EMS systems in which endotracheal intubation is medically approved, that approach to airway management should be considered for all comatose patients. Endotracheal intubation permits more certain control of the airway, facilitates ventilation of victims, and provides protection against aspiration of vomitus.

Upper-Airway Injury

Rapid onset of upper-airway injury leading to laryngeal edema, laryngospasm, airway obstruction, and asphyxiation can follow high-concentration inhalation exposure to water-soluble irritant gases. As described in chapter 15, such injury is most often associated with gases such as chlorine, ammonia, and hydrogen chloride. Response to upper-airway obstruction usually requires advanced-level airway management skills including endotracheal intubation or cricothyroidotomy. In this setting, endotracheal intubation can be especially difficult because chemical burns and edema will often greatly alter the normal airway anatomy.

If victims with signs of upper-airway obstruction cannot be intubated, because the EMS system operates at a basic life support (BLS) level or technical difficulties make it impossible to perform the intubation, then victims must be rapidly transported to a hospital or other definitive medical care facility. Few if any EMS systems permit prehospital cricothyroidotomy or other invasive airway maneuvers.

Excessive Secretions

Large volumes of fluid secretions can collect in the posterior pharynx and upper airway of exposure victims, which can lead to airway compromise. Highly reactive irritant chemicals, such as ammonia and chlorine, produce rapidly evolving burns of the upper airway. Large amounts of fluid move from the burned tissues into the airway. Fluid accumulation is also due to neurological poisons, particularly organophosphates and related insecticides, which provoke copious amounts of salivation and airway secretions.

In these victims, regular use of suction can help to maintain a patent airway. Consider endotracheal intubation (when medically approved) for victims with excessive secretions owing to airway burns. In victims without evidence of neck or spinal injuries, it is helpful to turn the victim's head to the side during suctioning.

Care must be taken to avoid injury of the soft tissues of the victim's mouth and throat during suctioning, especially with victims who have suffered chemical burns of those tissues. Burned tissues can be easily torn or punctured by forceful jabbing and sticking, or prolonged contact with the suction catheter.

AIDS TO BREATHING

Respirations and breathing may be decreased or absent in victims of hazardous chemical exposure. This can be due to severe CNS depression, coma, and respiratory paralysis. Exposure to solvents and other chemicals with strong anesthetic properties are a common cause. Highly lethal enzyme poisons such as cyanide and hydrogen sulfide can also produce respiratory paralysis. In addition, toxic exposure to cardiac sensitizers and agents that disturb electrolyte balance can cause cardiac arrest with associated apnea.

Victims who have suffered deep anesthesia must be immediately ventilated in fresh air and supplemental oxygen. Most will recover completely if effective respirations and cardiac output are maintained. It is also necessary to assure adequate ventilation in victims of cardiac arrest and enzyme poisons. Ventilation alone, however, is unlikely to lead to recovery in these patients.

Rescuers must take special precautions to avoid being contaminated when providing assisted ventilation to exposure victims. Mouth-to-mouth rescue breathing poses several specific risks. Some chemicals, such as hydrogen cyanide, are exhaled by exposure victims. Rescuers who perform mouth-to-mouth ventilation can inhale the chemical from the victim's breath and become poisoned. Because of this risk, *mouth-to-mouth ventilation should not be performed on victims of cyanide and related chemicals* such as the cyanide-containing compounds known as nitriles and cyanohydrins.

Rescuers can also suffer burns of the mouth or face if they perform mouth-to-mouth rescue breathing on victims who have suffered facial exposure to strong acids or alkali. Rescuers can also be burned by direct contact with the saliva or mucous membranes of victims who have suffered high-dose inhalation exposure to highly irritating, water-soluble chemicals such as ammonia, chlorine, or sulfur dioxide. Avoid direct contact with the contaminated skin and membranes of victims exposed to corrosives and other highly irritating chemicals until thorough decontamination has occurred.

In general, rescuers should use a bag-valve-mask when providing assisted ventilation to toxic exposure victims. If that equipment is not available, a pocket face mask provides some protection to rescuers performing mouth-to-mask ventilation. Besides providing protection to rescuers, bag-valve-masks and pocket face masks with an oxygen inlet allow victims to receive supplemental oxygen during assisted ventilation.

Supplemental oxygen is appropriate for most toxic exposure victims. In those who are alert and breathing, oxygen should be delivered according to the established protocols of the EMS system. In most cases, a nonrebreather face mask will be used. High concentrations of supplemental oxygen are essential for victims of exposure to asphyxiants and enzyme poisons. This point is especially true for victims of carbon monoxide and other chemicals that interfere with the blood's ability to carry oxygen. Victims of irritant inhalations and others who complain of shortness of breath or respiratory distress should also receive supplemental oxygen.

SUPPORT OF CIRCULATION

Hypotension and circulatory collapse can follow exposure to toxic chemicals that interfere with the body's control of the heart or vascular system. Examples of chemical-induced mechanisms producing circulatory collapse include the following:

1. Severe CNS depression can disrupt the vascular reflexes, which normally help to maintain the blood pressure.
2. Chemical-induced vasodilation and severe hypotension can be caused by agents such as phosphorus and nitrites, and other agents that act directly on blood vessels.
3. Cardiac dysrhythmias can be caused by exposure to toxic chemicals. For example, organophosphates and related insecticides can cause severe bradycardia and shock. Solvents that sensitize the heart to catecholamines can cause tachydysrhythmias and vascular collapse.
4. Allergic reactions and anaphylaxis can follow toxic exposure to chemicals such as formaldehyde and sulfur dioxide. Victims can suffer circulatory collapse and anaphylactic shock.
5. Fluid loss and hypovolemia leading to shock may result from severe chemical burns that allow fluids to leak out of blood vessels and into injured tissues.

All exposure victims must be closely monitored. The blood pressure and pulse should be determined frequently. In EMS systems that provide only BLS care, patients with evidence of hypotension or hypovolemia should be managed according to existing shock protocols. If possible, pneumatic antishock garments should be applied and then inflated as directed by medical control.

In EMS systems that provide advanced life support (ALS) care, intravenous infusions with Ringer's lactate or normal saline should be started in victims suspected of severe toxic chemical exposure. If no evidence of hypotension or hypovolemia exists, intravenous lines (IVs) should infuse at a to-keep-open rate. If hypotension, hypovolemia, or severe skin burns are present, then more aggressive infusion is necessary as directed by medical control. If physical examination findings such as crackles or rales suggest that pulmonary edema is actually present, then IVs should be maintained with D_5W (dextrose and water) rather than saline or Ringer's lactate.

EMERGENCY EYE PROCEDURES

Prompt and continuous irrigation with water or saline is the single most important aspect of caring for chemically exposed eyes. Some rescuers carry eye irrigation sets or irrigation contact lenses for this purpose. When washing the eyes, irrigating fluid should be poured gently into the nasal (medial) side of the eyes so that it flows out along the cheeks as shown in Figure 13–1.

An intravenous setup can be used to infuse either saline or Ringer's lactate into the eyes gently. This is useful in both the ambulance and the emergency department (Figure 13–2). In some cases, both eyes require simultaneous irrigation. Some rescuers manage these cases by placing a nasal oxygen canula over the bridge of the nose with nasal prongs pointing down toward the eyes. By attaching the canula to an intravenous setup, saline or Ringer's lactate can run continually into both eyes at once (Figure 13–2). If there is neither an eye irrigation set nor an intravenous setup available, a rubber bulb syringe taken from an obstetrics kit can be used to apply the irrigating fluid.

Irrigation lenses are useful for prolonged eye lavage in adults who do not have edema, lacerations, or penetrating wounds of the globe or eyelids. These

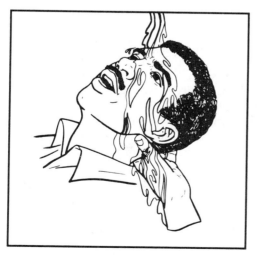

Figure 13–1 When irrigating the eyes, gently pour fluid into the nasal side of the eye so that it flows out along the cheeks.

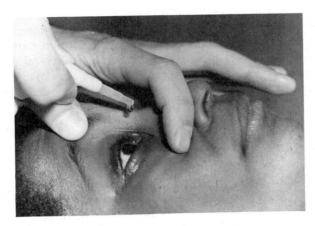

Figure 13–2 (a) Irrigation of the eye using normal saline and an intravenous setup. The eyelid is gently held open, and the saline is slowly dripped into the nasal side of the eye.

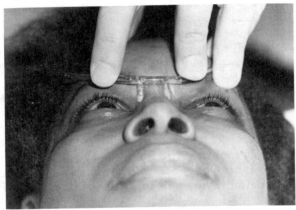

Figure 13–2 (b) Irrigating the eye by connecting an oxygen nasal canula to an intravenous setup allows a rescuer to irrigate both eyes simultaneously.

lenses permit continuous eye lavage without the continual presence of an emergency medical technician or other health care provider. Figure 13–3 demonstrates the insertion and removal of a Morgan Therapeutic Lens® (Mortan, Inc., Missoula, Montana). The lenses must be gently inserted to avoid causing additional trauma to the eye. These devices are not available in most EMS systems. They should be used only with medical approval.

Victims often resist prolonged eye irrigation. Reflexes stimulated by irritation and contact with the sclera and cornea cause a victim's eyelids to shut forcefully. This protective reflex makes irrigation difficult. To permit adequate washing, rescuers usually need to hold the eyelids open. When holding the eyelids open, pressure can be applied against the bony rim of the orbit but not against the eye itself.

Use of a topical anesthetic, when medically approved, minimizes the tendency for eyelid closure, facilitates prolonged eye irrigation, and permits insertion of irrigation lenses. One or two drops of a short-acting anesthetic such as pro-

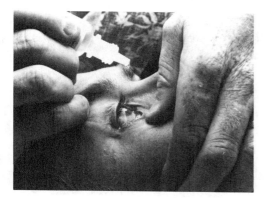

Figure 13–3a Instill topical anesthetic.

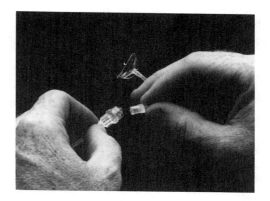

Figure 13–3b Attach syringe of intravenous set using solution and rate of choice; start flow.

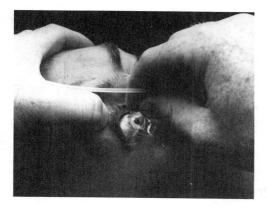

Figure 13–3c Have patient look down; insert lens under upper eye lid. Have patient look up; retract lower lid, and drop lens in place.

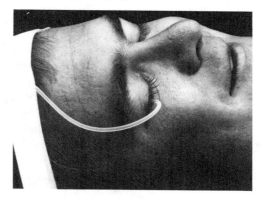

Figure 13–3d Release the lower lid over lens and continue flow. Tape the tube and adaptor to patient's forehead to prevent accidental lens removal. Absorb outflow with towels.

paracaine or tetracaine provides rapid-onset ocular anesthesia for 20 minutes to 1 hour. Before applying these agents, victims should be questioned about a history of allergy to caine-type anesthetics. Application of these agents can lead to severe allergic reactions in sensitized persons.

Topical ocular anesthetics are not currently approved in most EMS systems. Their use should be considered, however. These agents pose little risk to patients and facilitate the management of chemical eye exposure victims. They should not be used by emergency medical technicians or paramedics in systems that have not approved their use or without orders from a medical control physician.

For most chemical eye exposures, eye irrigation should be carried out for

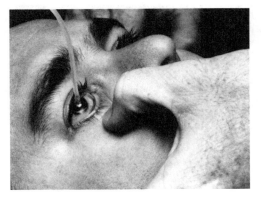

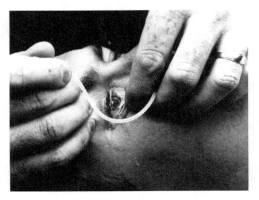

Figure 13–3e Removal: Have patient look up; retract lower lid, and hold position.

Figure 13–3f Slide the lens out.

at least 15 minutes. After alkali exposures, at least 20 minutes of irrigation is necessary. When possible, irrigation after alkali and acid exposures should be continued until the conjunctival sac pH approaches values in the normal range (normal pH of 6 to 8). A simple technique for measuring the conjunctival pH is shown in Figure 13–4. If the conjunctival pH cannot be measured, then irrigation should be continuously carried out until the victim has been transported to a definitive medical care facility.

Rescuers should be certain that no foreign bodies or solid particles of chem-

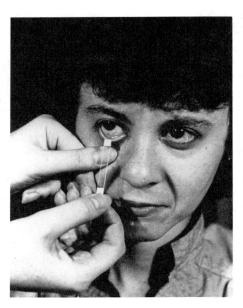

Figure 13–4 To measure the conjunctival sac pH using a urine pH dipstick, the lower lid is gently pulled down, and the pH-sensitive strip is touched right against the conjunctiva. This can also be performed with litmus paper or other pH paper. (Slide no. 8, ''Ophthalmology for ER Staff,'' reprinted with permission, American Academy of Ophthalmology.)

icals are on the eye or under the eyelids. Such materials can increase the damage caused to the eye. Examination must be made under both eyelids. A technique for examining under the eyelids is shown in Figure 13–5. If foreign materials are present on the underside of an eyelid and cannot be washed away, they should be gently removed with a sterile, moist cotton tip swab. Emergency medical technicians and paramedics should not attempt to remove foreign bodies from the cornea except by washing them away.

The presence of contact lenses can contribute to the severity of injuries following chemical eye exposures. Contact lenses should be removed promptly when possible. Lens removal should be performed carefully to avoid causing further injury to the cornea. It may be necessary to use a lens removal suction bulb. If a contact lens cannot be easily removed, however, slide it away from the iris onto the sclera and continue washing the eye.

It is important to remember that the eye is especially fragile after alkali burns. Rough handling or excessive pressure can cause its surface to be torn and perforate. To protect the eye, it should be touched and handled as little as possible while the victim is transported to a definitive medical care facility.

EMERGENCY SKIN PROCEDURES

Chemical skin exposures can lead to localized skin burns, percutaneous absorption, and systemic poisoning. The goal of emergency management is to remove contaminating chemicals from the skin as quickly as possible. In most cases, that is accomplished by washing the skin with water or soap and water.

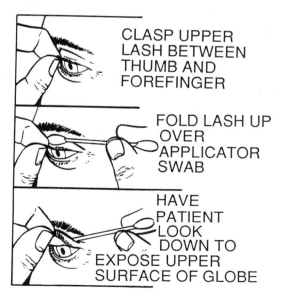

CLASP UPPER LASH BETWEEN THUMB AND FOREFINGER

FOLD LASH UP OVER APPLICATOR SWAB

HAVE PATIENT LOOK DOWN TO EXPOSE UPPER SURFACE OF GLOBE

Figure 13–5 Removing a foreign object from the eye. Clasping the lash with the thumb and forefinger, fold the lash over the applicator swab. Never attempt to remove an object on the cornea.

The victim's clothing, shoes, and jewelry must be removed. Prolonged contact with contaminated clothing can produce severe exposure reactions. For example, contact with clothing soaked by ethylene oxide produces severe skin burns. Contact with clothing wet by nitriles can lead to percutaneous absorption and fatal cyanide poisoning. Some chemicals, such as organophosphates and related insecticides, are well absorbed by leather from which they are slowly released. People who wear leather products can suffer intoxication.

The importance of promptly washing contaminated skin and continuing for at least 15 minutes is emphasized in chapter 17 (see Table 17–1). Most chemical plants and factories have emergency showers. The initial washing of victims will have begun before the arrival of EMS personnel. In other settings, however, adequate washing facilities may not be available. Washing can be carried out by using a shower, garden hose, bathtub or pouring buckets of water over the victim. The stream of water used should be continuous but gentle so that burned tissues are not further injured.

Most EMS systems emphasize rapid transport of all victims. It may be useful in such systems to develop specific protocols for chemical burn victims to encourage a minimum of 15 minutes of skin washing before transport. This protocol is appropriate for all exposure victims who have not suffered some other life-threatening emergency.

Water soluble chemicals can usually be washed adequately with water alone, but fat-soluble chemicals require washing with soap or mild detergent and water. If rescuers are in doubt about the identity of a specific chemical or its solubility, then a soap or detergent wash should be performed.

In most cases, following skin washing, victims should be covered with dry, sterile dressings, or burn sheets, and rapidly transported to a definitive medical care facility. After alkali burns, however, use of wet dressings with continuous irrigation is more appropriate. Wet compresses are also appropriate for phosphorus burns, as described later.

Water washing is necessary for the treatment of almost all chemical skin exposures *except* contamination by alkali metals. Examples include sodium, lithium, and dry calcium salts such as lime and portland cement. Those metals and calcium salts react with water to produce heat and alkaline solutions that can severely injure the skin. Dry lime and portland cement should first be brushed off the skin and then a wash with large amounts of water can be used. Alkali metals should not be water washed. They should be covered with mineral oil or some other light oil to prevent air contact with the metal during transport to a medical care facility.

Some chemicals require unique or specialized skin care procedures. Several will be described in more detail in chapter 17. *Phosphorus*, for example, ignites spontaneously at temperatures above 86°F. Exposure victims, therefore, require skin cooling of the involved area. During transport, cool wet compresses should be applied to the skin. *Phenol* (carbolic acid) is a corrosive substance that is only slightly water soluble. It is best removed from the skin by washing first with polypropylene glycol (or an alcohol) and then with water. *Hydrogen fluoride* (hydrofluoric acid) can cause severe skin injuries because of its effects upon the calcium salts of the body. In addition to water washing, exposure victims require replacement of calcium as described later (see section on antidotes). In communities where these and other "special" chemicals are known to be routinely used, EMS planners should consider developing specific patient management protocols.

Rescuers must be careful to avoid becoming contaminated by contact with chemicals on the skin of victims. When possible, they should wear at least double latex or vinyl gloves. Care must also be taken by rescuers to avoid splashing themselves or others with the run-off of water used to wash contaminated victims. The use of liquid-resistant protective clothing such as polyethylene-coated material coveralls can protect EMS personnel performing skin washing.

EMERGENCY CARDIAC PROCEDURES

Cardiac emergencies that can develop in victims of hazardous chemical exposures include the following:

1. Cardiac dysrhythmias

2. Cardiac arrest

3. Pulmonary edema

These emergencies may result from the direct effects of toxic chemicals on the heart and lungs. They can also be secondary events, as when chemical exposure leads to myocardial infarction in an exposure victim with underlying coronary artery disease.

All exposure victims must be closely monitored. In EMS systems that provide ALS care, electronic cardiac monitors should be used for victims who have been exposed to chemicals known to disrupt or alter the cardiac rhythm. Examples of such chemicals include the following:

1. *Organophosphate and related insecticides* can cause severe bradycardia and heart block leading to asystole.

2. *Organic solvents* (such as toluene) and *halogenated hydrocarbons* (such as trichloroethylene) can sensitize the heart to epinephrine. They promote the development of tachydysrhythmias including ventricular tachycardia and fibrillation.

3. *Anesthetic agents* (such as ethyl chloride) can produce various types of heart blocks leading to ectopic ventricular contractions. Both asystolic and ventricular fibrillation can result.

4. *Asphyxiants* produce myocardial ischemia and can cause rhythm distur-

bances associated with myocardial infarction and coronary artery disease. Hydrogen cyanide and related chemicals have been associated with various types of heart block.

5. *Sequestration agents* (such as hydrogen fluoride, oxalic acid, and phosphorus) can cause severe hypocalcemia, which can lead to prolongation of the QT interval of the electrocardiogram, ventricular ectopic beats, and cardiac arrest.

6. *Alkaline metals* such as sodium, potassium, and lithium can be absorbed leading to electrolyte disturbances associated with dysrhythmias, heart blocks, and cardiac arrest.

7. *Pulmonary irritants* provoke vagus nerve reflexes that result in bradycardia and hypotension. Inhalation exposure severe enough to cause pulmonary edema often causes myocardial ischemia. Rhythm disturbances associated with myocardial infarction and coronary artery disease can result.

In EMS systems that operate at the ALS level, rhythm disturbances should be treated by standard paramedic cardiac protocols. Standard medication dosages may not be appropriate, however. For example, victims of exposures to solvents and other cardiac-sensitizing chemicals should generally receive less than standard doses of epinephrine, dopamine, norepinephrine, and isoproterenol when any of those catecholamines are required. By contrast, bradycardia and heart block owing to organophosphate insecticide exposure is likely to require doses of atropine that are much greater than those routinely used for cardiac patients.

Pulmonary edema developing after inhalation of chemicals is rarely due to heart failure. As described more fully in chapter 15, edema develops as a result of increased lung permeability and loss of the lung's normal protective mechanisms. Edema can develop immediately after inhalation exposure or its onset can be delayed for hours or longer.

The physical examination is not an adequate means of distinguishing between victims with cardiogenic pulmonary edema and those with permeability pulmonary edema. Unfortunately, some pulmonary edema treatments that are useful for heart failure patients can worsen the condition of inhalation victims. Diuretics, for example, are often used in heart failure to increase urine production and decrease blood volume. In patients with permeability pulmonary edema, who may have normal or low blood volumes, the use of diuretics can lead to hypovolemia, decrease cardiac output, and cause cardiac failure.

Pulmonary edema from inhalation exposures is much less common than cardiac edema. For that reason, and because these two types of patients cannot be distinguished by clinical examination, EMS systems should not develop special protocols for inhalation pulmonary edema. Such patients should be treated by standard pulmonary edema protocols. EMS responders must be particularly careful, however, in managing inhalation victims because standard cardiac protocols may cause them harm.

Patients with pulmonary edema should receive supplemental oxygen. These patients may be more comfortable sitting up with their arms and legs in dependent positions. Airway management should include suctioning of secretions.

In EMS systems that provide ALS care, endotracheal intubation and positive pressure ventilation may be necessary for adequate oxygenation of severe edema victims. Commonly used ALS medications (such as diuretics, morphine, and aminophylline) may have only limited or even negative effects on permeability pulmonary edema. When administering those medications by standing orders, paramedics should consider giving doses that are as small as protocols allow. Consultation with a medical control physician is advised to determine the appropriate uses and doses of medications.

ANTIDOTES

Antidotes are medications or agents that block or reverse the effects of poisons. Only a few antidotes are useful for victims of hazardous chemicals. Still fewer antidotes can be administered safely by EMS personnel. In most cases, prehospital use of antidotes requires specific protocols or orders given by a medical control physician. The use and actions of several antidotes of value in prehospital care are described subsequently.

Organophosphate Insecticides

Organophosphate and carbamate insecticides are nerve poisons. Exposure victims develop excessive activity of the parasympathetic nervous system. This problem leads to a characteristic clinical syndrome including bradycardia, hypotension, heart block, and respiratory failure with asthma. The full syndrome will be described in chapter 18.

Antidotal management of these victims involves blocking the parasympathetic hyperactivity. Two commonly used medications for this purpose are atropine and pralidoxime (PAM). Because the effects of organophosphate insecticides can be rapid and severe, antidotal treatment must often be started as quickly as possible. Except when specific protocols with standing orders have been developed, these treatments require the orders of a medical control physician.

Initial treatment involves administration of large intravenous doses of atropine. In adults, an initial atropine dose of 2 to 4 mg has been recommended with similar doses repeated every 5 to 10 minutes until the insecticide's effects have been blocked. In children, doses of about 0.05 mg per kg have been recommended. Adequate amounts of atropine have been administered when the lungs of victims are clear to auscultation, excessive salivation and lacrimation have ceased, and pupils have become dilated.

Following successful atropinization, pralidoxime is then administered. This medication is not routinely carried by EMS personnel and will rarely be available for prehospital administration.

The total dose of atropine required to reverse the effects of an organophosphate poisoning fully can be huge. There has been at least one report of a successfully treated victim who received more than 3900 mg of atropine and 90 g of pralidoxime during a treatment period that lasted more than 3 weeks.

Cyanide and Hydrogen Sulfide

Hydrogen cyanide, hydrogen sulfide, and related cyanide compounds are lethal enzyme poisons. Both cyanide and sulfide act by binding to metal atoms in the enzymes that they poison. Their lethal effects are due to the ability to bind to and block *cytochrome oxidase,* an enzyme that is critical for cellular respiration. Blocking cytochrome oxidase prevents cells from using oxygen and causes cellular anoxia.

The goal of antidotal treatment is to remove the cyanide or sulfide from cytochrome oxidase so that the enzyme can resume function. This is done by providing other metal atoms to which cyanide and sulfide are strongly attracted. The standard antidotal approach in North America involves agents that oxidize the iron atoms of hemoglobin from the ferrous (Fe^{+2}) state to the ferric (or Fe^{+3}) state and thereby transform hemoglobin into methemoglobin. Cyanide and sulfide are more strongly attracted to methemoglobin than to cytochrome oxidase.

Methemoglobin is usually produced by administering nitrites. The necessary medications are packaged together in Lilly Cyanide Antidote Package (Figure 13–6). These medications should not be used without medically approved protocols or orders from a medical control physician. Initially, amyl nitrite perles are broken and placed under the victim's nose or over the bag-valve-mask intake

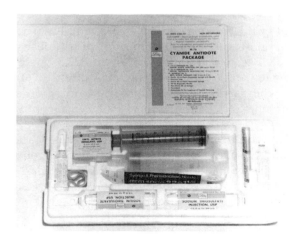

Figure 13–6 The cyanide antidote kit should be available to all emergency departments and personnel. All medications currently used as antidotes and administration supplies are included in one package.

port for 15 to 30 seconds of every minute. Then, a 3 percent solution of sodium nitrite is prepared and 10 to 15 ml are infused intravenously for 4 to 5 minutes. Amyl nitrite perles can produce a methemoglobin level of about 5 percent, whereas nitrite infusions can produce levels in excess of 30 percent. Pediatric doses are presented in Table 13–1.

Cyanide victims should also receive infusions of sodium thiosulfate (50 ml of a 25 percent solution IV for 10 minutes). This helps the body to transform cyanide to a harmless substance, thiocyanate, which is excreted in the urine. Pediatric doses are presented in Table 13–1. Thiosulfate administration is not required for sulfide poisoning.

Antidotal use of nitrites can be effective even in patients who are unconscious and apneic. They are potentially dangerous, however. Because methemoglobin cannot transport oxygen, formation of excessive methemoglobin can result in fatal tissue anoxia. Also, infusions of nitrites can cause extreme hypotension. Treated patients must be closely monitored. If hypotension develops, large amounts of intravenous fluids or pressor agents such as dopamine may be required to restore blood pressure.

Because of the toxicity of nitrites and also the difficulty in diagnosing cyanide poisoning on clinical grounds, most EMS systems do not include cyanide antidotes as protocol medications. In some systems, amyl nitrite perles can be used for suspected cyanide and hydrogen sulfide victims while patients are rapidly transported to hospitals or other definitive medical care facilities.

A safer antidote, hydroxocobalamin (vitamin B_{12A}), has been successfully used for cyanide poisonings in Europe and is under investigation in the United States. This vitamin attracts cyanide from cytochrome oxidase and binds with it to form harmless cyanocobalamin (vitamin B_{12}). Because hydroxocobalamin can be administered without risk of side effects, it is likely that it will become the

TABLE 13–1 PEDIATRIC DOSES OF CYANIDE ANTIDOTES*

	IV dose (ml/kg)	
Hemoglobin level	3% Na[+] nitrite	25% Na thiosulfate
7	0.19	0.95
8	0.22	1.10
9	0.25	1.25
10	0.27	1.35
11	0.30	1.50
12[†]	0.33[‡]	1.65[‡]
13	0.36	1.80
14	0.39	1.95

*Berlin, 1970.

[†]Average pediatric dose.

[‡]Na = sodium.

standard treatment for cyanide exposures. It may be employed as a medication in EMS systems that provide ALS care.

Hydrogen Fluoride

Hydrogen fluoride and its water solution, hydrofluoric acid, are potent acids that are also damaging because of their ability to lower blood and tissue levels of calcium. Management of skin burn victims requires the use of antidotal agents that replace calcium and remove fluoride from the tissues.

A simple approach that can be carried out by EMS personnel involves a calcium gluconate gel rubbed into the exposed skin. Such gels are not commercially available, but they can be easily made by mixing 2.5 g of calcium gluconate USP in 100 ml of a water soluble lubricant such as Surgilube® (Altana, Inc., Melville, N.Y.) or KY Jelly® (Johnson and Johnson Patient Care, New Brunswick, N. J.). Following water washing of the burned skin, the gel is massaged continuously into the burned area until pain is relieved or the patient has been transported to a definitive medical care facility. A rubber, vinyl, or latex glove should be used to protect the hand used to massage the gel.

A suitable calcium gel is often available at industrial sites where hydrogen fluoride is routinely used. EMS systems in areas where hydrogen fluoride exposures are common should consider the development of specific protocols for the preparation and use of the gel by EMS personnel. Few if any side effects can result from this treatment.

If pain has not been relieved after 30 minutes of continuous application of calcium gluconate gel, then more aggressive administration of calcium is usually required. This approach can be accomplished by injecting aqueous calcium gluconate into and around the burn site. Burns of the fingers and toes may require infusions of calcium into the arteries of the hand or foot. These techniques are not generally performed by EMS personnel.

The onset of pain may immediately follow exposure to concentrated acid or it can be delayed up to 24 hours after exposure to dilute concentrations. Once pain develops, however, its persistence is an important criterion for judging the success of antidotal treatment. The presence of pain is an indication that treatment has not yet been adequate. Exposure victims should not receive anesthetics or other pain medications. Suppressing the pain limits the ability to monitor the adequacy of treatment.

Oxygen

Oxygen is not generally thought of as an antidote for poisoning victims, but it can function as one. For example, oxygen has important value as an antidote for patients exposed to carbon monoxide and methylene chloride. Those two chemicals produce dangerously high blood levels of carboxyhemoglobin. Because carboxyhemoglobin cannot transport oxygen in the blood, formation of high levels can cause fatal tissue anoxia.

After victims have been removed from exposure to carbon monoxide or methylene chloride, carboxyhemoglobin levels decrease slowly. In room air, the half-life of carbon monoxide-induced carboxyhemoglobin is greater than 4 hours. By contrast, the carboxyhemoglobin levels falls quickly when victims breathe 100 percent oxygen. The half-life in that case is less than 1 hour. Even more rapid clearing of carboxyhemoglobin occurs when victims are placed in hyperbaric oxygen chambers. At oxygen pressures of about 3 atmospheres, carboxyhemoglobin half-life is less than 30 minutes.

Administration of high concentrations of oxygen can prevent death or severe disability resulting from carbon monoxide or methylene chloride exposures. In victims suspected to have suffered these exposures, 100 percent oxygen should be administered through a tight-fitting nonrebreather face mask with high oxygen flow rates (at least 6 to 12 liters per minute). In unconscious patients, 100 percent oxygen should be supplied through an endotracheal tube when medically approved. For severely exposed victims, use of a hyperbaric oxygen chamber should be considered.

Some evidence indicates that hyperbaric oxygen also acts as an antidote for poisoning by carbon tetrachloride, an industrial solvent that causes liver, kidney, and lung injuries. Use of high concentrations of oxygen and hyperbaric treatments should be considered for severe exposure victims. Little or no evidence indicates that oxygen acts as an antidote for victims of cyanide or hydrogen sulfide. Hyperbaric oxygen has been used for victims of exposure to both, but the value of such treatments remains unproven.

SUMMARY

The prehospital care of hazardous materials exposure victims is based on standard EMS knowledge and procedures. Rescuers must assure that all victims have an open airway, adequate breathing, and circulation. Prompt and thorough washing of the eyes and skin are necessary for contaminated persons. Close monitoring of patients is also necessary. Exposure to hazards can lead to rapidly developing cardiac irregularities which must be recognized.

Only a few antidotes are of value to EMS systems. Rescue personnel should be familiar with these treatment methods, and EMS systems should consider medical approval and protocols for their use. Antidotal treatments should be provided only at the direction of a medical control physician.

REFERENCES

AMMANN, H. M., "New Look at Physiologic Respiratory Response to H$_2$S Poisoning." *J. Haz. Mat.*, 13 (1986), 369–74.

BAKINSON, M. A., and R. D. JONES, "Gassings due to Methylene Chloride, Xylene, Toluene, and Styrene Reported to Her Majesty's Factory Inspectorate, 1961–80,'' *Br. J. Ind. Med.*, 42 (1985), 184–90.

BASS, M., ''Sudden Sniffing Death,'' *JAMA*, 212 (1970), 2075–79.

BEAUCHAMP, R. O., J. A. POPP, C. J. BOREIKO, et al: ''Critical Review of the Literature on Hydrogen Sulfide Toxicity,'' *CRC Crit. Rev. Toxicol.*, 13 (1984), 25–97.

BERLIN, C. M., ''The Treatment of Cyanide Poisoning in Children,'' *Pediatrics*, 46 (1970), 793–96.

BLEDSOE, B. E., G. BOSKER, and F. J. PAPA, *Prehospital Emergency Pharmacology*. Bowie, Md.: Brady Communications Company, Inc., 1984.

BOWEN, T. E., T. J. WHELAN, and T. G. NELSON, ''Sudden Death after Phosphorus Burns: Experimental Observations of Hypocalcemia, Hyperphosphatemia and Electrocardiographic Abnormalities following Production of a Standard White Phosphorus Burn,'' *Ann. Surg.*, 174 (1971), 779–84.

BROADDUS, V. C., Y. BERTHIAUME, J. W. BIONDI, M. A. MATTHAY, ''Hemodynamic Management of the Adult Respiratory Distress Syndrome,'' *J. Intensive Care Med.*, 2 (1987), 190–213.

BRONSTEIN, A. C., and P. L. CURRANCE, *Emergency Care for Hazardous Materials Exposure*. St.Louis: The C. V. Mosby Company, 1988.

CLARK, R., ''Ocular Emergencies,'' in *Emergency Medicine*, pp. 581–88. eds., J. E. Tintinalli, R. L. Krome, and E. Ruiz. New York: McGraw-Hill Book Company, 1988.

CUMMINGS, C. C., and M. E. MCIVOR, ''Fluoride-Induced Hyperkalemia,'' *Am. J. Emerg. Med.*, 6 (1988), 1–3.

CUSHMAN, P., and B. H. ALEXANDER, ''Renal Phosphate and Calcium Excretory Defects in a Case of Acute Phosphorus Poisoning,'' *Nephron*, 3 (1966), 123–28.

DIBBELL, DAVID G., RONALD E. IVERSON, WALLACE JONES, et al: ''Hydroflouric Acid Burns of the Hand,'' *J. Bone Joint Surg.*, 52A (1970), 931–36.

ELLENHORN, M. J., and D. G. BARCELOUX, *Medical Toxicology*. New York: Elsevier North-Holland, Inc., 1988.

EMMETT, E. A., ''Toxic Responses of the Skin,'' in *Casarett and Doull's Toxicology: The Basic Science of Poisons*, pp. 412–31, eds. C. D. Klaassen, M. O. Amdur and J. Doull. New York: Macmillan Publishing Co., Inc., 1986.

ENGER, E., ''Acidosis, Gaps and Poisonings'' [editorial], *Acta Med. Scand.*, 212 (1982), 1–3.

GOLDFRANK, L. R., and R. M. KIRSTEIN, ''Cyanide: Cyanogenic Glycosides,'' in *Goldfrank's Toxicologic Emergencies* (3rd ed.), pp. 585–97, eds. L. R. Goldfrank, N. E. Flomenbaum, N. A. Lewin, et al. Englewood Cliffs, N.J.: Prentice Hall, Inc., 1986.

GOLDFRANK, L. R., N. A. LEWIN, R. H. KIRSTEIN, R. S. WEISMAN, ''Carbon Monoxide,'' in *Goldfrank's Toxicologic Emergencies* (3rd ed.), pp. 662–71, eds. L. R. Goldfrank, N. E. Flomenbaum, N. A. Lewin, et al. Englewood Cliffs, N.J.: Prentice Hall, Inc., 1986.

GOLDFRANK, L. F., E. A. BRESNITZ, R. H. KIRSTEIN, M. A. HOWLAND, "Organophosphates," in *Goldfrank's Toxicologic Emergencies* (3rd ed.), pp. 686–96, eds. L. R. Goldfrank, N. E. Flomenbaum, N. A. Lewin, et al. Englewood Cliffs, N.J.: Prentice Hall, Inc., 1986.

GRANT, H. D., R. H. MURRAY, J. D. BERGERON, *Emergency Care*. Englewood Cliffs, N.J.: Prentice Hall, Inc., 1986.

GRANT, W. M., *Toxicology of the Eye*. Springfield, Ill.: Charles C Thomas, 1986.

HALL, A. H., and B. H. RUMACK, "Clinical Toxicology of Cyanide," *Ann. Emerg. Med.*, 15 (1986), 1067–73.

KIZER, K. W., "Hyperbaric Oxygen and Cyanide Poisoning," *Am. J. Emerg. Med.*, 2 (1984), 113–18.

MCLAUGHLIN, R. S., "Chemical Burns of the Human Cornea." *Am. J. Ophthalmol.*, 29 (1946), 1355–62.

MENCHEL, S. M., and W. A. DUNN, "Hydrofluoric Acid Poisoning," *Am. J. Forensic Med. Pathol.*, 5 (1984), 245–48.

MENZEL, D. B., and M. O. AMDUR, "Toxic Responses of the Respiratory System," in *Casarett and Doull's Toxicology: The Basic Science of Poisons*, pp. 330–58, eds. C. D. Klaassen, M. O. Amdur, and J. Doull. New York: Macmillan Publishing Co., Inc., 1986.

MORGAN, D. P., *Recognition and Management of Pesticide Poisonings*. Washington, D.C.: U.S. Environmental Protection Agency, 1982.

MURPHY, S. D., "Toxic Effects of Pesticides," in *Casarett and Doull's Toxicology: The Basic Science of Poisons*, pp. 519–81, eds. C. D. Klaassen, M. O. Amdur, and J. Doull. New York: Macmillan Publishing Co., Inc., 1986.

NELSON, J. D., and L. A. KOPIETZ, "Chemical Injuries to the Eyes: Emergency, Intermediate, and Long-Term Care," *Postgrad. Med. J.*, 81 (1987), 62–75.

NORTON, S., "Toxic Responses of the Central Nervous System," in *Casarett and Doull's Toxicology: The Basic Science of Poisons*, pp. 359–86, eds. C. D. Klaassen, M. O. Amdur, and J. Doull. New York: Macmillan Publishing Co., Inc., 1986.

O'DONOGHUE, J. L., "Aliphatic Halogenated Hydrocarbons, Alcohols, and Acids and Thioacids," in *Neurotoxicity of Industrial and Commercial Chemicals* (vol. 2), pp. 99–126, ed. J. L. O'Donoghue. Boca Raton, Fla.: CRC Press, 1985.

O'DONOGHUE, J. L., "Alkanes, Alcohols, Ketones, and Ethylene Oxide," in *Neurotoxicity of Industrial and Commercial Chemicals* (vol. 2), pp. 61–97, ed. J. L. O'Donoghue. Boca Raton, Fla.: CRC Press, 1985.

O'DONOGHUE, J. L., "Aromatic Hydrocarbons," in *Neurotoxicity of Industrial and Commercial Chemicals* (vol. 2), pp. 127–37, ed. J. L. O'Donoghue. Boca Raton, Fla.: CRC Press, 1985.

POTTS, A. M., "Toxic Responses of the Eye," in *Casarett and Doull's Toxicology: The Basic Science of Poisons*, pp. 478–515, eds. C. D. Klaassen, M. O. Amdur, and J. Doull. New York: Macmillan Publishing Co., Inc., 1986.

RALPH, R. A., and H. H. SLANSKY, "Therapy of Chemical Burns," in *Practical*

Management of Ocular Injuries, pp. 171–91, ed. S. A. Boruchoff. Boston: Little, Brown & Company, 1974.

REINHARDT, C. F., A. AZAR, M. E. MAXFIELD, et al: "Cardiac Arrhythmias and Aerosol 'Sniffing'," *Arch. Environ. Health,* 22 (1971), 265–79.

REINHARDT, C. F., L. S. MULLIN, and M. E. MAXFIELD, "Epinephrine-Induced Cardiac Arrhythmia Potential of Some Common Industrial Solvents," *J. Occup. Med.,* 15 (1973), 953–55.

SMITH, R. P., "Toxic Responses of the Blood," in *Casarett and Doull's Toxicology: The Basic Science of Poisons,* pp. 223–44, eds. C. D. Klaassen, M. O. Amdur, and J. Doull. New York: Macmillan Publishing Co., Inc., 1986.

TANII, H., and K. HASHIMOTO, "Structure-Acute Toxicity Relationship of Dinitriles in Mice," *Arch. Toxicol.,* 57 (1985), 88–93.

TEPPERMAN, PAUL B., "Fatality due to Acute Systemic Fluoride Poisoning Following a Hydrofluoric Acid Skin Burn," *J. Occup. Med.* 22 (1980), 691–92.

VANCE, M. V., S. C. CURRY, D. B. KUNKEL, et al: "Digital Hydrofluoric Acid Burns: Treatment with Intraarterial Calcium Infusion," *Ann. Emerg. Med.,* 15 (1986), 890–96.

WAY, J. L., "Cyanide Intoxication and Its Mechanism of Antagonism," *Ann. Rev. Pharmacol. Toxicol.,* 24 (1984), 451–81.

WRIGHT, P., "Chemically Injured Eye," *Trans. Ophthalmol. Soc. UK,* 102 (1982), 85–87.

PROTECTION OF THE HEALTH CARE SYSTEM

CHAPTER 14

GOAL: On completion of this chapter the student will have an understanding of the importance of protecting the "downstream" health care system and the procedures to be followed to guard against contamination.

OBJECTIVES:

Specifically the student will be able to

- Name the people and things in the health care system requiring protection, and discuss the importance of protection for each
- Discuss the ways in which EMS personnel can be protected from contamination by hazardous materials
- Describe the procedures for protecting EMS equipment and vehicles from contamination by hazardous materials
- Describe the procedures for protecting the emergency department and its staff from contamination by hazardous materials
- Discuss the kinds of protective equipment and supplies that are needed for ambulance-based EMS personnel to protect themselves and their ambulances

OVERVIEW

This chapter describes some procedures and preplanning issues that can help protect the health care system and its personnel from contamination during hazardous materials incidents. Emergency responders involved at an incident should be constantly aware that risk of exposure and injury exists. Moreover, it should be understood that rescuers and incident victims are not the only ones at risk. Contamination can be transmitted "downstream" from the site of the original incident. As a result, contamination can spread to involve other rescuers, rescue equipment and vehicles, and even the hospital and its emergency department to which victims are transported.

To protect themselves, rescuers should take care to avoid unnecessary exposures and to use appropriate personal protective equipment when entering contaminated places. Protecting the downstream health care system requires that rescuers carefully perform decontamination and follow other incident safety procedures. In addition, a need exists for preplanning so that personnel, ambulances and hospital facilities can be adequately protected from contamination.

GOAL

The goal of protecting the downstream health care system is to prevent contamination of health care workers and the facilities in which they work. By avoiding contamination, it is possible to assure that all facilities and personnel will continue to function and provide care to the community's sick and injured. A real danger exists that personnel, ambulances, hospitals, or emergency departments may be unable to function and provide care if they are not protected from contamination.

Protection should be provided to all personnel, equipment, and facilities that are involved in caring for victims of hazardous materials exposure. Those who might become contaminated through incidental contact with victims, personnel, or equipment should also be protected. The following partial list of people and things make up the emergency health care system and require some protection:

1. EMS personnel

2. EMS vehicles and equipment

3. Emergency department personnel

4. Emergency department patients

5. Emergency department facility

6. Hospital

When EMS or emergency department personnel become contaminated by hazardous chemicals, they risk personal illness. In addition, a possibility exists that they will pass the contamination along to their patients, colleagues, and others. When EMS equipment and vehicles become contaminated, a risk exists that the equipment will be out of service until decontamination has been completed. Sometimes, equipment or vehicles cannot be decontaminated and must be destroyed. Contamination of the emergency department or other areas of the hospital may require that those areas be closed to patients until decontamination has been completed.

A contaminated health care system threatens the health and well-being of health care workers. Moreover, that health care system can lose its ability to provide needed services. Such an event can cause much greater hardship than was caused by the hazardous material incident that created the emergency in the first place.

PROTECTION OF EMS PERSONNEL

EMS personnel, like other emergency responders who work at the actual site of a hazardous material incident, are at risk of contamination. The risk can be minimized by limiting the number of personnel who have access to the contaminated area, assuring that appropriate protective equipment is used, and enforcing careful decontamination of all personnel and equipment. Some specific guidelines and procedures to provide such protection are described subsequently.

Restriction of Access to the Contaminated Area

Only the fewest possible rescue personnel should be allowed to enter zones of high contamination. EMS personnel should not be allowed to enter contaminated areas for reasons other than victim assessment or rescue.

Limitation of Number of Involved Personnel

A natural tendency exists for crowds to form at the scenes of accidents and disasters. Even among rescuers, attraction and fascination with the disaster can lead to unnecessary crowding. Unlike most other types of accidents, however, hazardous materials can affect and harm observers and bystanders. For this reason, the number of EMS personnel involved at an incident should be limited to the fewest actually needed. Surplus personnel should remain at a staging site distant from the area of contamination.

Protect Pregnant Staff

A great deal is not known about the effects that most acute chemical exposures have on fetuses. Enough suspected harm exists, however, to argue that pregnant women should not be allowed to enter an area of chemical contamination. The purpose of this guideline is to protect the unborn child from potential toxic harm.

PROTECTING EMS PERSONNEL

1. Restrict access
2. Limit number of personnel
3. Pregnant women should not be involved
4. Decontaminate all exposed personnel
5. Use appropriate CPC
6. Ventilate ambulance during transport
7. Maintain personal exposure log

Decontamination of All Exposed Personnel

Any emergency responder who becomes exposed to harmful chemicals must undergo decontamination. In the excitement of responding to an industrial accident, EMS personnel must not neglect their own decontamination.

Appropriate Use of Personal Protective Equipment

EMS personnel must not enter heavily contaminated areas without proper personal protective equipment. The choice of personal protective equipment should be based on identification of the contaminating chemicals and determination of their environmental concentrations.

Personnel who do not actually enter the incident hot zone, but who have physical contact with potentially contaminated victims, should also be protected from becoming contaminated. Those rescuers should at least consider use of disposable chemical protective clothing, and latex or vinyl gloves. A list of protective equipment and supplies that should be carried in an ambulance or rescue vehicle is presented later.

Ventilation of Ambulance during Transport

A danger always exists that residual contamination remains on a victim, rescuers, or rescue equipment. When contaminated victims or rescuers are in the unventilated patient compartment of an ambulance, dangerous concentrations of chemicals can develop. Exposure of victims and EMS personnel can occur, and EMS responders may suffer exposure injury. In these cases, the ambulance should be ventilated while the victim is being transported to hospital. Ventilation should be maintained whenever the ambulance crew is uncertain about the adequacy of decontamination.

Maintenance of Personal Exposure Log

Emergency responders involved in hazardous materials incidents should keep a diary that records all exposures and contaminations that they have suffered. The diary should include names of chemicals causing exposure, dates of the exposures, and any symptoms that developed. In addition, responders should undergo regular, periodic medical examinations and routine laboratory testing. The information contained in the exposure log should be made available to the responder's personal physician at the time of medical examinations.

Medical surveillance, described more fully in Appendix 4, involves periodic medical examinations of workers who are regularly exposed to high levels of hazardous chemicals. Medical surveillance must also be provided to workers who develop symptoms as a result of toxic exposures. Many employers are required by federal regulations to provide medical surveillance examinations to their employees who work with hazardous materials. Unfortunately, most emergency responders and EMS personnel do not fit into the groups of workers for whom periodic examinations are required.

Response personnel who anticipate exposure to hazardous materials should have a complete physical examination before beginning emergency response work ("preplacement examination"), an annual physical examination, an examination at the termination of response work ("exit examination") and an examination following each documented hazardous material exposure. The purpose of these examinations is to recognize intoxication promptly when it occurs and to assure that workers receive appropriate medical care when needed. A written report for each examination should be included in the personal exposure log.

PROTECTION OF EMS EQUIPMENT AND VEHICLES

Victims of hazardous materials exposure who are transported in an ambulance or other EMS vehicle can contaminate that vehicle and its equipment. This is especially likely when victims with severe injuries and need for rapid transport to a health care facility are transported after only superficial decontamination. Once contaminated, an ambulance may not be usable until decontamination has been performed. The vehicle may be out of service for days or longer.

This potential problem can be avoided by a small effort and proper planning. A simple, seven-step approach to protecting an ambulance from contamination follows.

> **PROTECT EQUIPMENT
> AND VEHICLES**
>
> 1. Set aside needed equipment
> 2. Remove unnecessary equipment
> 3. Tape ambulance compartments
> 4. Encapsulate patient compartment
> 5. Return needed equipment to ambulance
> 6. Use disposable and portable equipment
> 7. Monitor contamination

1. *Identify and set aside needed equipment:* The ambulance equipment that will likely be needed for patient care should be removed from the vehicle and set aside. This should include equipment and supplies that are normally stored in drawers and lockers in the patient compartment. This equipment will be returned to the ambulance shortly.

2. *Remove unnecessary equipment:* Transporting vehicles often carry equipment that will not be needed during a hazardous materials incident such as stair chairs and extra stretchers. This equipment should be removed and stored for later use (Figure 14–1).

3. *Tape closed all ambulance compartments:* Once all necessary equipment has been removed from the ambulance drawers and lockers, those compartments should be sealed closed with duct tape. If the vehicle is equipped

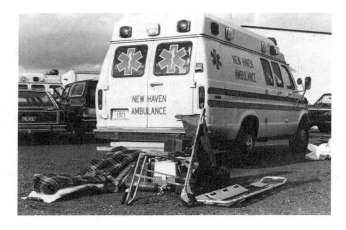

Figure 14–1 All nonessential and portable equipment should be removed from the transporting vehicle.

with a storage locker under the bench seat, the doors of that locker should also be taped shut. The tape should be applied so that the compartments and storage areas are sealed closed from the patient compartment. Figure 14–2 illustrates the sealing of storage compartments.

4. *Encapsulate the patient compartment:* The inside of the patient compartment should be encapsulated by heavy gauge plastic or Tyvek sheets that are taped to the four sides of the compartment. Sheets should be taped from the ceiling to the floor on each wall and along the front of the patient compartment. A sheet of plastic or a fire department salvage tarpaulin should be placed on the compartment floor with the edges rolled to create a catchment basin for water or other contaminants. If possible, a plastic sheet should be taped to the ceiling as well. Figure 14–3 illustrates an ambulance being prepared in this way to transport hazardous materials exposure victims.

   The radio, main oxygen supply, and suction equipment will now have been sealed behind plastic sheets and will not be available to the patient compartment. Portable equipment should be used for treatment at the scene and during transport.

5. *Return all needed equipment to ambulance:* The equipment that will be needed to care for victims and that was removed earlier from the ambulance

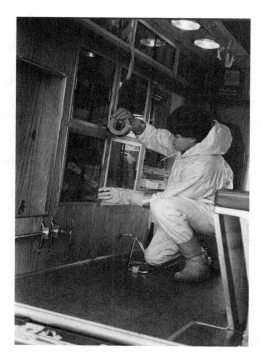

Figure 14–2 The cabinet doors are being sealed with heavy-duty plastic sheets and heavy duct tape.

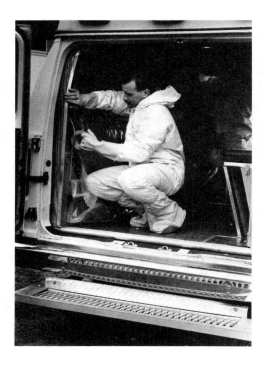

Figure 14–3 Sheets of heavy-duty plastic are draped along the ambulance walls and are secured with heavy duct tape.

should now be returned to the patient compartment. This equipment is placed within the plastic covered area in which patients will be treated.

6. *Use disposable and portable equipment:* Whenever possible, use portable or disposable equipment for treating hazardous materials victims. This suggestion will make decontamination of equipment as easy as possible and will avoid loss of a major vehicle if a component piece of equipment becomes contaminated.

7. *Monitor contamination:* After victims have been transported to the emergency department, it is recommended that the vehicle and crew return to the hazardous material incident for decontamination. If the ambulance will not be needed for additional exposure victims, the plastic and tape should be removed and disposed of in an area designated for contaminated wastes and materials. The vehicle should be monitored and decontaminated if necessary (Figure 14–4). The crew should go through decontamination to the extent required by their level of contamination and exposure.

PROTECTIVE EQUIPMENT AND SUPPLIES

A minimum amount of protective equipment and supplies are needed so that ambulance-based EMS personnel can protect themselves and their ambulances. The equipment listed subsequently is appropriate for ambulance crews who re-

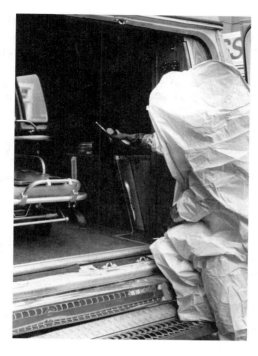

Figure 14–4 The transporting vehicle is monitored for contaminants.

main outside of heavily contaminated areas. It is also appropriate for rescue personnel who care for victims who have received incomplete decontamination. Rescuers who are exposed to higher levels of contamination require higher levels of personal protection.

1. *Gloves* should be worn by all rescuers who have physical contact with exposure victims. Generally, use of double layers of vinyl or latex surgical gloves provide adequate protection when victims have undergone decontamination. A large supply of vinyl or latex examining gloves should be available in the ambulance.

    If rescuers are likely to care for heavily contaminated victims, then higher levels of glove protection should be considered. Use gloves that are made of materials effective against the chemicals to be encountered. Rescuers should refer to compatibility charts when selecting the glove to use at a hazardous materials incident. Such compatibility charts are usually provided by glove manufacturers. Compatibility charts are also available in reference books such as *Guidelines for the Selection of Chemical Protective Clothing.*

    When special protective gloves are worn by rescuers, vinyl or latex gloves should also be worn as an inner lining. These higher-protection gloves tend to be thick and clumsy. They can interfere with hand dexterity and sensitivity of touch. Wearing them will restrict the ability of rescuers to perform delicate EMS procedures. They may also limit the ability of a rescuer to perform a secondary survey.

    Specific types of commonly used chemical protective gloves are described subsequently. They are listed from least expensive to most expensive. Also presented are general recommendations about the classes of chemicals for which each provides good or bad protection. Because many exceptions to these recommendations exist, rescuers should verify the appropriateness of each type of glove before it is used.

- *Natural rubber* gloves are flexible and inexpensive. They offer only limited protection, however. They are useful for protection against alcohols and dilute acids and bases. They offer poor protection against most organic chemicals and solvents.
- *Nitrile rubber* gloves provide good general purpose protection. These gloves are relatively flexible and inexpensive. They are good protection against alcohols, oils and fuels, alkali, amines, and phenols. They are poor protection against aromatic and halogenated hydrocarbons, amides, ketones, and esters.
- *Neoprene rubber* gloves offer good protection against strong alkali, dilute acids, alcohols, phenols, fuels and oils, and aliphatic hydrocarbons. They are not protective against aromatic and halogenated hydrocarbons, ketones, and concentrated acids. They are several times more expensive than nitrile rubber gloves.
- *Butyl rubber* gloves are effective protection against alkali and many organic chemicals, but they are not protective against aliphatic, aromatic, or halogenated hydrocarbons or gasoline. They are nearly twice as expensive as neoprene rubber gloves.
- *Viton* gloves provide good protection against organic solvents (such as aliphatic, aromatic and halogenated hydrocarbons, and acids). They do not provide protection against ketones, esters, aldehydes and amines. They are more than ten times more costly than nitrile and neoprene rubber gloves.

2. *Overboots* of latex or neoprene should be worn on the feet to protect rescue personnel from contamination caused by water run-off and other spilled liquids.

3. *Face shields* or *safety goggles* should be worn to prevent splash exposure of a rescuer's eyes, nose, or mouth. Shields and goggles also protect against contamination by dusts. Equipment of this type does not protect against inhalation of toxic gases.

4. *Chemical resistant jumpsuits* can protect rescue personnel from exposures resulting from liquids and dusts. Some suits can also protect EMS personnel from exposure to blood and other body fluids. In general, laminated suits offer more resistance than nonlaminates. Examples of suitable protective fabrics include Tyvek® (The DuPont Company, Wilmington, Del.) coated with either polyethylene or Saranex® (The Dow Chemical Company, Midland, Mich.).

Protective suits that are disposable are usually least expensive. Suits should have hoods. Keep available either a selection of sizes or only extra-large sizes to be certain that suits will fit all personnel.

5. *Sheets* of plastic or Tyvek® in sufficient size should be available so that the inside of the ambulance can be encapsulated.

6. *Duct tape* should be available.

7. *Stretchers* should be used that do not absorb hazardous materials. For example, metal or plastic stretchers are adequate. Stretchers with cloth, wood, or leather parts will absorb chemicals and pose a risk of contamination to future victims and rescuers.

8. *Reference books* should be available to EMS personnel who must research the health effects of specific hazardous materials exposures. A list of appropriate books and reference sources is provided in chapter 5.

PROTECTION OF THE EMERGENCY DEPARTMENT AND ITS STAFF

It is important that the emergency department and hospital to which exposure victims are transported not become contaminated. If contamination did occur, it might be necessary for the entire hospital or its emergency department to be closed until decontamination had been completed. The emergency department staff and any patients who happen to be in the emergency department must also be protected.

The following guidelines and procedures describe some ways to avoid contamination of the emergency department facility and its staff when hazardous materials exposure victims are transported to hospital.

1. *Perform triage outdoors:* When possible, triage and assessment of victims should occur outside of the hospital and its emergency department. The fewer the number of contaminated patients who enter the emergency department and the more slowly they enter, the more likely that contamination can be controlled. It is possible that some triaged patients will not require admission to the emergency department and that others can receive further decontamination before emergency department entry (Figure 14–5).

2. *Use a separate emergency department entrance:* Potentially contaminated victims should enter the emergency department through a separate hazardous materials entrance that leads them to an area where decontamination and assessment can be performed (Figure 14–6). In this way, it is less likely that other patients and public areas will be contaminated.

3. *Use a designated treatment room:* Victims should be fully decontaminated be-

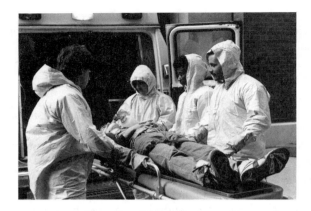

Figure 14–5a The rescuers and hospital personnel, dressed in jumpsuits to avoid possible contamination, lower the victim from the ambulance.

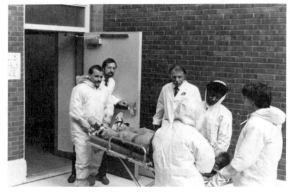

Figure 14–5b Emergency department medical personnel come out to the transporting vehicle to greet the rescuers and guide the rescue team through the hazardous materials emergency entrance.

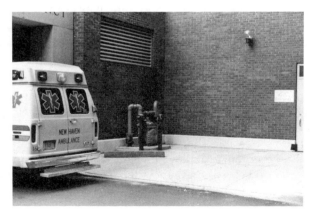

Figure 14–6 Whenever possible, a separate entrance to the emergency department should be used when transporting victims of hazardous emergencies.

fore they are allowed to enter the open emergency department. If contaminated patients need emergency care before complete decontamination, they should be evaluated and treated in designated areas that are not simultaneously used by other patients (Figure 14–7).

If possible, these rooms should be closed, self-contained spaces to

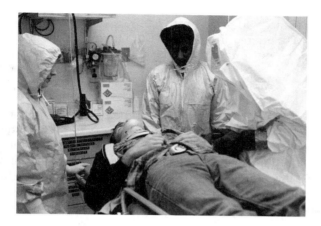

Figure 14–7 Use a designated treatment room.

limit the spread of contaminants further. The room should be clearly marked so that hospital staff are warned of contamination dangers. Exposure victims should not be allowed to make contact with other patients who happen to be in the emergency department at the same time.

PROTECTION OF EMERGENCY DEPARTMENT

1. Perform triage outdoors
2. Use separate entrance
3. Use designated treatment room
4. Restrict access
5. Limit staff contact
6. Use CPC
7. Protect emergency department from contaminants
8. Maintain personal exposure log
9. Monitor cleanup
10. Isolate drainage and ventilation

---

4. *Restrict access to treatment room:* Only personnel directly involved in the care of exposure victims should be allowed to enter the treatment area. Visitors and guests must not be permitted to visit these patients until all contamination risks have been addressed.

5. *Limit staff contact with exposure victims:* The number of emergency depart-

ment staff who have contact with exposure victims should be limited to the minimum number actually required. Those staff members should not have responsibility to other uncontaminated patients who happen to be in the emergency department at the same time. Pregnant staff members should not be assigned to care for victims of hazardous chemical exposures.

6. *Consider use of personal protective equipment:* Even in the emergency department, the use of personal protective equipment can serve to protect staff from contamination. Disposable Level B jumpsuits provide relatively inexpensive protection of staff members performing triage and decontamination of patients. Double layers of vinyl or latex gloves can also be used for additional staff protection.

7. *Protect emergency department from contaminants:* The floor over which exposure victims and rescuers travel should be covered with heavy gauge plastic sheets so that contaminants do not make contact with the emergency department floor. Disposal bags and barrels should be available to contain victims' clothing and other contaminated materials.

8. *Maintain a personal exposure log:* All emergency department staff who have direct contact with hazardous materials or hazardous materials victims should keep a diary in which they record all exposures or contaminations that they have suffered. The diary should include the names of chemicals that caused exposure, the date of the exposure, and any symptoms that develop. In addition, responders should undergo regular, periodic medical examinations and routine laboratory testing. The information contained in the exposure log should be made available to the responder's personal physician at the time of each medical examination.

   Any staff member who has suffered a documented hazardous materials exposure should have a medical examination directed to the possible effects of that exposure. A written report of the examination findings should be included in the personal log.

9. *Monitor cleanup:* After exposure victims have been treated and either discharged or transferred, the emergency department treatment rooms should be monitored to assure that no residual contamination is present before those rooms are used for other patients.

10. *Isolate drainage and ventilation:* When possible, exposure victims should be washed and treated in hospital areas that have water drains leading to isolated holding tanks and ventilation systems that are independent of those used by the rest of the hospital. Unfortunately, these concerns have only rarely been addressed in the design and construction of hospitals. As a result, the wash water in many hospitals is drained into community sewer systems, and a risk often exists that airborne contaminants will be carried throughout the hospital via ventilation systems.

   One way to contain contaminated wash water effectively is by use of

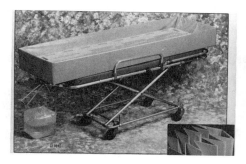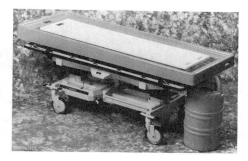

Figure 14–8   Two examples of commercial decontamination stretchers with self-contained collection systems. (Courtesy of Radiation Management Consultants, Philadelphia, Pa.)

a decontamination stretcher with hosing that drains the water into a self-contained collection system or into a reservoir or 55-gallon drum (Figure 14–8). A morgue table can be readily turned into a decontamination stretcher for this purpose.

SUMMARY

Emergency responders involved with hazardous materials incidents must help to protect the downstream health care system from contamination. Their goal should be to assure that the entire health care system continues to function properly despite the presence of hazardous chemicals. To achieve that goal, it is necessary to restrict the spread of contamination. Protection must be provided to EMS personnel, EMS vehicles and ambulances, emergency department staff and patients, and the physical facility of the emergency department and hospital. The protocols and guidelines presented earlier provide methods for protecting the various components of the health care system.

REFERENCES

BRONSTEIN, ALVIN C., and PHILLIP L. CURRANCE, *Emergency Care for Hazardous Materials Exposure*, St. Louis: The C. V. Mosby Company, 1988.

CARLSON, GENE P., ed., *HazMat Response Team Leak and Spill Guide*. Stillwater, Okla.: Fire Protection Publications, 1984.

Guidelines for the Selection of Chemical Protective Clothing. Cambridge, Mass.: Arthur D. Little, 1987.

Hazardous Materials Response for First Responders. Washington, D.C.: U.S. Environmental Protection Agency, 1987.

Proceedings of "The Medical Management of HazMat Incidents," presented by Michael S. Hildebrand, American Petroleum Institute, and Prince George Fire Department's Hazardous Materials Response Team; sponsored by the EMS degree program, George Washington University, Washington, D.C., June 1988.

NOLL, GREGORY G., MICHAEL S. HILDEBRAND, and JAMES G. YVORRA, *Hazardous Materials: Managing the Incident.* Stillwater, Okla.: Fire Protection Publications, 1988.

PHYSIOLOGY OF TOXIC INHALATION INJURIES

CHAPTER 15

GOAL: On completion of this chapter the student will have an understanding of the ways that inhaled chemicals can injure the lung and will be able to describe the properties of those chemicals that determine the type and location of injuries suffered.

OBJECTIVES:

Specifically, the student will be able to

- Describe how a knowledge of the physical properties, chemical properties, and physical form of a hazardous chemical can be used to predict the likely type and location of lung injury that will result
- List five factors in an exposure victim's prior condition that help to determine whether inhalation of a hazardous material will cause lung injury
- Describe the types of chemicals that are likely to cause upper-airway injury following inhalation and the kinds of injuries that may develop
- List four major effects of inhaled chemicals that can lead to obstruction of the bronchioles
- Describe the ways that inhaled chemicals can provoke asthma attacks
- Explain the differences between pulmonary edema caused by inhalation of chemicals and cardiogenic pulmonary edema

OVERVIEW

This chapter focuses on the acute lung injuries that result from inhalation of harmful chemicals. First, the anatomy and architecture of the lung will be reviewed as related to toxic inhalation. Next, some factors will be examined that determine the type and severity of lung damage. The most important of those factors include the properties of the specific chemicals that have been inhaled and the baseline condition of the inhalation victims. Finally, some commonly encountered types of inhalation lung injuries will be discussed.

This chapter will not be concerned with chemicals that are absorbed from the lungs. Those chemicals that cause systemic poisoning after being absorbed will be considered in chapter 18.

Our lungs are exposed to harmful chemicals with almost every breath we take. The air of the industrialized world contains chemicals that come from fires, motor exhaust fumes, and industrial processes. Toxic fumes and gases can be inhaled as we work at jobs that range from farming to mining to chemical manufacture. Even in homes and schools many are concerned about the health effects of inhaled toxins like asbestos and radon. Inhalations such as these generally cause health effects only after exposure of many years. Rarely do such inhalations cause acute medical emergencies.

Under other circumstances, immediate lung injury can result from even brief toxic inhalation, which is usually due to the effects of high concentrations of reactive chemicals. In such settings, life-threatening injury may evolve rapidly. Exposures of this type are usually caused by industrial accidents and are almost never due to "normal" air pollution.

ANATOMIC CONSIDERATIONS

It is useful to first consider the architecture of the human respiratory system (Figure 15–1). Inhaled air initially passes through the *nasopharynx*. As described in chapter 9, the hair and cilia of the nasal passages can remove toxic chemicals from inhaled air before it reaches the lungs. Mouth breathing is less effective than nose breathing for removing airborne chemicals. Greater amounts of inhaled toxins reach the airways and alveoli of mouth breathers.

The *airways* of the lung begin at the larynx as a single large tube, the trachea, and terminate as millions of tiny tubules, the alveolar ducts, that open into the alveoli. Between the trachea and the alveoli, the airways branch more than twenty times. The largest of the branching airways are called *bronchi*. As they grow smaller they are called *bronchioles*. Finally, when hardly larger than the alveoli, the tubules are called *alveolar ducts* (Figure 15–2).

As the bronchioles branch, the diameter of the individual tubules become narrower, the number of tubules increases greatly, and the total cross-sectional area of the airways becomes large. Between the bronchi and the alveoli, a two-thousand–fold increase in the cross-sectional area of the airways exists. This branching sequence of the airways is illustrated in Figure 15–3.

Air flows rapidly through the bronchi and large bronchioles, like water cascading downhill. In the smallest bronchioles and alveolar ducts, conversely,

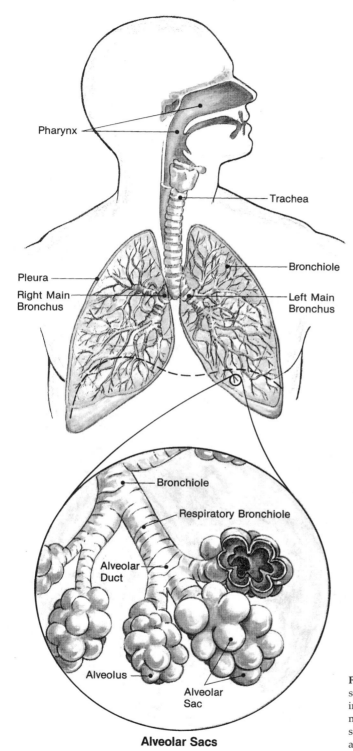

Figure 15–1 The human respiratory system consists of airways that direct inhaled air to the gas-exchange membranes of the alveoli. The main structures of the respiratory system are indicated here.

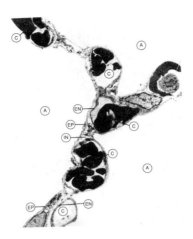

Figure 15–2a Electron microscopic picture of the alveolar membranes (A = alveolus; C = capillary; EP = alveolar epithelial cell; EN = capillary endothelial cell). (Courtesy of G. J. Walker Smith, M.D., Yale University School of Medicine, New Haven, Conn.)

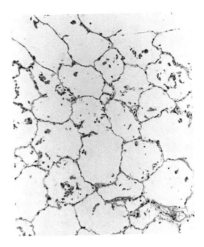

Figure 15–2b Light microscopic picture of the alveoli showing the thin alveolar membranes (A = alveolus; EP = alveolar epithelial cells). (Courtesy of G. J. Walker Smith, M.D., Yale University School of Medicine, New Haven, Conn.)

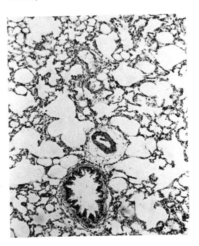

Figure 15–2c Light microscopic picture of alveoli surrounding the small bronchiole and pulmonary capillary (A = alveolus; B = bronchiole; C = capillary). (Courtesy of G. J. Walker Smith, M.D., Yale University School of Medicine, New Haven, Conn.)

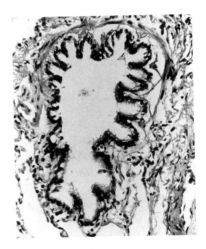

Figure 15–2d Microscopic picture showing a bronchiole in high magnification. (Courtesy of G. J. Walker Smith, M.D., Yale University School of Medicine, New Haven, Conn.)

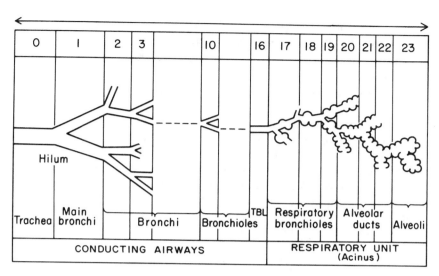

Figure 15–3 A schematic rendering of the human airways as they branch from the trachea to the alveoli. (Adapted from Weibel, E. R., *Morphometry of the Human Lung,* p. 3. Heidelberg: Springer-Verlag, [1963].)

air flows slowly like the movement of water in a river delta or swamp. Inhaled dust and other foreign material tend to be carried by the in-rushing of air down to the small airways where particles settle.

The airways are lined with specialized cells that secrete mucus along the airway surface. Other cells have cilia, fine hairlike structures that extend from the cell borders and sweep accumulated mucus out of the lung. The mucus tends to trap and remove inhaled chemicals. For example, dust particles stick to mucus and are swept away by the cilia. In a similar way, water-soluble gases dissolve in the surface water, mucus of the nasopharynx, and airways, and are removed from the inhaled air before reaching the alveoli.

The *alveoli* are tiny air sacs that make up the lung's gas-exchange membrane. In a normal person, about 300 million alveoli are in each lung. The alveolar membrane is thin and delicate, only about one cell thick. It has a large surface area, however: In an average-sized adult, that membrane's size is between 500 and 1,000 square feet.

Alveoli are lined by two kinds of cells. Type I cells are flat and thin, and cover about 97 percent of the alveolar surface. Type II cells are small and round, and represent more than half of all alveolar cells, but cover only 3 percent of the alveolar surface. The primary function of type II cells is to secrete *surfactant,* a fatty substance that plays an important role in keeping alveoli functional. Both cell types are essential for successful breathing (see Figure 15–2).

It is useful to think of the lung as having three separate anatomic regions.

1. The *conducting airways* are the largest of the airway tubes. They include the trachea, bronchi, and larger bronchioles.
2. The *respiratory bronchioles* are the smallest of the airway tubules. They connect the larger bronchioles to the alveoli.
3. The *alveoli* represent the gas-exchange membranes of the lung.

Different types of chemical exposures will affect these regions differently. Chemicals that are soluble in water tend to cause injury to the conducting airways. Chemicals that are not water soluble tend to injure the alveoli. Conducting airway injuries can lead to rapid asphyxia because they become blocked. Alveolar injury can produce pulmonary edema, often delayed in onset, that may be fatal. Irritation of the respiratory bronchioles can produce asthmalike disorders.

PROPERTIES OF CHEMICALS

The type and location of injury caused by an inhaled chemical depends on the specific actions and behaviors of that chemical. Those actions and behaviors can be categorized according to three types of chemical factors.

1. Physical properties
2. Physical form
3. Chemical properties

Physical Properties

The *concentration* of a chemical in air helps to determine the severity of inhalation injury. At low concentrations, many chemicals are removed from inhaled air before reaching the respiratory bronchioles and alveoli. At higher concentrations, conversely, large amounts can penetrate into the lungs, causing extensive lung damage.

The *duration of exposure* is nearly as important as the concentration. For any given chemical concentration, prolonged exposures will lead to more lung injury than briefer exposure. Prolonged exposure to a low concentration is sometimes more harmful than brief exposure to high concentrations.

The *exposure dose* is determined by both the chemical concentration and the exposure duration:

$$Dose = Concentration \times Duration$$

Increasing either the concentration or the duration increases the dose received by an exposed victim. Most chemicals have ''dose-related effects,'' meaning that the amount of injury caused is related to the dose that was inhaled.

The *solubility* of a chemical in water is a measure of how much and how quickly that chemical dissolves in water. Soluble chemicals are likely to dissolve in the moisture coating the mucous membranes of the nasopharynx and conducting airways. Once dissolved, these chemicals can cause local injury. Water-soluble chemicals (such as ammonia and chlorine) can provoke severe damage to the moist membranes of the pharynx and upper airways. By contrast, insoluble chemicals (such as phosgene and nitrogen dioxide) have little toxic impact on the conducting airways but can severely damage the alveoli and respiratory bronchioles.

Physical Form

Chemicals can be inhaled as gases, mists, fumes, or particles. *Gases* and *vapors* mix with air and distribute themselves freely throughout the lung and its airways. *Mists* consist of liquid droplets dispersed in air. The size of mist droplets determine the severity of exposure effects. At higher humidity and temperature, droplet size tends to grow larger and exposure effects increase. *Fumes* contain fine particles of dust dispersed in air. The ability of fume particles to penetrate into the lung depends on particle size. Large particles are likely to be trapped in the nasopharynx and conducting airways. Small particles are more likely to penetrate deeply to the respiratory bronchioles and alveoli. The relationship between dust particle size and site of deposit after inhalation is shown in Figure 15–4.

Chemical Properties

The *reactivity* of a chemical refers to its ability to interact with other chemicals and body tissues. Generally, highly reactive chemicals cause severer and more rapid injury than less reactive chemicals.

The *pH* of a chemical is a measure of its ability to react as an acid (low pH) or as an alkali (high pH). As the pH of an acid falls or the pH of an alkali increases, a greater likelihood of severe injury following exposure exists. Strong

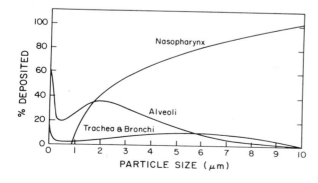

Figure 15–4 Relationship of particle size (mass median diameter) to deposition sites in the respiratory system. (From Hollinger, M. A., *Respiratory Pharmacology and Toxicology*, p. 169. Philadelphia: W. B. Saunders Company, [1985]; reprinted with permission.)

acids (pH less than 2) and strong alkali (pH greater than 11.5) can cause massive tissue destruction.

Some chemicals are *direct acting,* that is, they are able to cause harm without first being transformed or changed. *Indirect acting* chemicals must be transformed before they can provoke injury. The difference between direct and indirect acting chemicals can be illustrated by comparing the toxic effects of hydrogen chloride and phosgene. These two gases have similar toxic mechanisms, but they affect different parts of the lung.

Hydrogen chloride is an acid that is direct acting and extremely water soluble. After inhalation, hydrogen chloride gas dissolves in the surface water and mucus of the upper airways, and can cause severe acid burns. Alveolar injury is rare, however, because little of the inhaled hydrogen chloride actually reaches the alveoli except after massive exposure.

Phosgene, by contrast, is an extremely hazardous gas that is water insoluble. It can cause injury by several mechanisms of which one involves its conversion to form hydrogen chloride, a process that may require several hours. Most of an inhaled phosgene dose can reach the alveoli where hydrogen chloride is then formed and results in acid burns of the alveolar membranes.

Another type of injury is caused by some reactive chemicals that bind with proteins to form structures that stimulate allergic mechanisms. Chemicals with high allergic potential, such as formaldehyde, can cause severe asthmatic and anaphylactic reactions after even small exposures. In general, the allergic potential of a chemical is related to its reactivity.

It is important to note that some chemicals can cause severe clinical injury even though they are not very reactive. One classic example is lead, a metal that is used to insulate nuclear reactors because it is so nonreactive. Nevertheless, lead can cause severe injury to those who are exposed both acutely and chronically.

CONDITION OF VICTIM

Whether inhalation exposure leads to illness or injury is determined in part by the victim's condition before that exposure. Of importance are the following factors:

1. The rate and pattern of respirations

2. History of previous lung disease

3. Victim's age

4. Victim's nutrition

5. Victim's thyroid function

The *rate and pattern of respirations* influence the development of inhalation injury. Hyperventilation and mouth breathing both allow greater amounts of inhaled toxins to reach the lungs. When greater amounts of chemicals reach the lungs, greater damage and injury can be expected.

Persons with a history of *previous lung disease* are more likely to suffer serious reactions after acute inhalation exposure and after smaller inhaled doses. These people include cigarette smokers, asthmatics, and those with chronic lung diseases (such as bronchitis and emphysema).

The *age* of a victim can influence the effects of exposure. Some chemicals, particularly oxidant gases such as ozone and nitrogen dioxide, cause greater injury in older people than in the young.

The status of a victim's *nutrition* is also important. Malnutrition leads to deficiencies of proteins and vitamins that normally protect the body against chemical exposures. Two examples are vitamin E and glutathione. Large doses of vitamin E have been used to treat victims of oxygen toxicity as well as inhalation victims of other oxidizing agents. In laboratory experiments, animals deprived of vitamin E are particularly vulnerable to lung injury owing to oxidant gases.

Glutathione is a sulfur-containing protein that is normally found in large quantities in the liver and lungs. It can block the toxic effects of numerous types of chemicals including oxidants, vesicants, alkylating agents, and other harmful and toxic agents. Malnutrition leads to glutathione deficiency and increased risk of toxic lung injury. Figure 15–5 demonstrates the increased toxic effects of an inhaled alkylating agent, measured in terms of the amount of covalent binding caused by that agent, as the level of lung glutathione falls.

Like nutritional status, a victim's *thyroid function* also affects vulnerability to inhalation injury. Low thyroid function (hypothyroidism) leads to increased lung concentrations of glutathione and, as just described, protection against inhalation injury. Increased thyroid function (hyperthyroidism), conversely, makes victims more vulnerable to inhalation injury by decreasing lung glutathione levels.

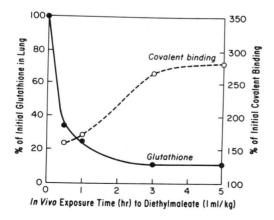

Figure 15–5 Effect of glutathione depletion on binding to lung protein by an inhaled alkylating agent. (From Hollinger, M. A., S. N. Giri, and F. Hwang, ''Binding of Radioactivity from ^{14}C-Thiourea to Rat Lung Protein,'' *Drug Metab. Dispos.*, 4 [1976], 121.)

INHALATION INJURY TO UPPER AIRWAY

The conducting airways are easily injured by inhaled chemicals that are *water soluble* and very *reactive*. Examples include acids (such as chlorine and hydrogen chloride), alkali (such as ammonia), and vesicants (such as formaldehyde). As these chemicals are inhaled, they dissolve in the moisture that coats the airways and cause intense inflammation and chemical burns.

Massive laryngeal edema and laryngospasm can develop rapidly after severe exposure to such chemicals. These problems can lead to obstruction of the upper airways, asphyxia, and death. Less severe exposure leads to bronchitis, laryngitis, and tracheitis.

Airway obstruction and laryngeal edema must be considered a possibility in every inhalation victim, especially after exposure to water-soluble gases. Emergency responders must evaluate the victim's pattern of respirations and determine the presence of *stridor*. Stridor is a harsh, high-pitched respiratory sound that occurs during inhalation, heard through a stethoscope placed over the throat rather than lungs. Victims must be closely observed and regularly reassessed because respiratory distress can develop suddenly, even hours after exposure. Aggressive airway management, including endotracheal intubation (when medically authorized), can be life saving for these victims.

BRONCHIOLAR OBSTRUCTION AFTER INHALATION INJURY

Injury to the lower conducting airways and terminal bronchioles comes about when chemicals penetrate more deeply into the lung. It can occur with chemicals that are not very water soluble, when the chemical is inhaled at a high concentration, or when exposure has been prolonged.

Four major effects of chemicals on the bronchioles are as follows:

1. Narrowing owing to local edema

2. Obstruction owing to sloughed airway cells

3. Disruption of cilia

4. Obstruction owing to pooled secretions

Edema is the most immediate effect. It results from injury to the airway lining cells and disruption of deeper airway tissues.

Necrosis of cells can occur rapidly. Necrotic cells then separate from the airway walls and fall into the bronchiolar lumen, a process known as *sloughing*. Ulcerations and sterile abscesses of the bronchioles can evolve. After severe exposure, the entire airway lining can slough as a single sheet of tissue that looks like a "cast" of the bronchus.

Exposure can lead to obstruction of the smaller airways. Following chemical injury, the airway cells lose their cilia. As damage to cilia becomes severe, the airways lose their ability to clear away mucus, secretions, and cell debris.

Small amounts of secretions and mucus are normally present in the airways. After chemical injury, however, secretions increase in quantity and become thick and sticky. Mixed with the debris of sloughed cells, the thick mucus secretions collect in the bronchioles and clog them. This most often occurs in airways that have also suffered loss of cilia. In those airways, clearing of the bronchioles is more difficult than in healthy airways.

Bronchiolar obstruction can occur immediately after exposure or be delayed for hours or longer. In some cases, severe exposure causes symptoms that are similar to asthmatic attacks. Others may seem more like pulmonary edema. Victims complain of chest discomfort. Cough is often prominent. Increased lung sounds (especially wheezes) usually are audible, and the expiratory phase of the breathing cycle may be prolonged (Figure 15–6).

BRONCHOSPASM

Some toxic chemicals can provoke classic asthma attacks in victims of inhalation exposure, even when the exposure dose is small. Those chemicals may act as typical allergens, substances that provoke allergic reactions.

Many people have been sensitized to industrial chemicals as a result of day-to-day contact. Most do not know that they have been sensitized, however, and are at risk. For example, formaldehyde is used in newspaper ink and wash-and-wear clothing. Contact with newspapers or clothing can lead to formaldehyde sensitization. Following inhalation of even low formaldehyde doses, sensitized persons can develop classic allergic asthma and other common allergic reactions.

Asthmatic reactions can begin immediately after exposure or onset may be delayed for up to 6 hours. The dose of chemical required to initiate severe asthma in a sensitized person is much less than that needed to cause lung injury in nonallergic, nonsensitized exposure victims. For example, sensitized people can develop severe asthmatic attacks after brief exposure to low formaldehyde concentrations. Nonsensitized people only develop similar symptoms after exposure to concentrations fifty times greater.

Asthmalike reactions can also occur for nonallergic reasons. Irritation of nerves in the membranes of the nasal passages cause reflex narrowing of terminal bronchioles and asthmalike complaints. Very reactive chemicals (such as acids, alkali, and vesicants) can cause this effect. Most people who develop these reactions, however, also have underlying asthma.

Asthmatic and asthmalike reactions to inhaled chemicals can be severe and can last for 48 hours or more. Patients complain of difficulty breathing, wheezes can be heard, the expiratory phase of breathing is prolonged, the pulse rate is often elevated, and coughing may be prominent. Some patients also complain of chest tightness or discomfort. Anaphylactic reactions can also occur. Victims with signs of asthma must be carefully observed, and vital signs must be reassessed regularly.

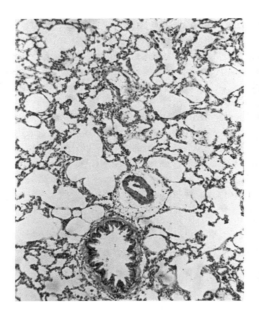 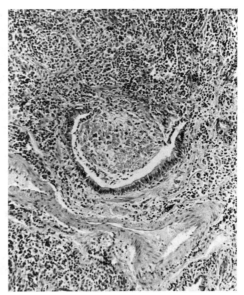

Figure 15–6a Light microscopic picture of normal bronchiole along with a neighboring capillary. (Courtesy of G. J. Walker Smith, M.D., Yale University School of Medicine, New Haven, Conn.)

Figure 15–6b Light microscopic picture of a bronchiole and capillary showing the effects of broncholitis obliterans, which nearly fills the bronchiolar lumen and has caused the capillary to collapse (B = bronchiole; C = capillary). (Courtesy of G. J. Walker Smith, M.D., Yale University School of Medicine, New Haven, Conn.)

PULMONARY EDEMA

Pulmonary edema can occur whenever inhaled chemicals cause damage to the alveoli. This is most likely to occur in the following situations:

1. Inhalation of irritating chemicals that are water insoluble

2. High-concentration inhalation exposure

3. Prolonged exposure

The normal lung has several mechanisms that protect against pulmonary edema. Interference with those protective mechanisms by inhaled chemicals causes edema. For example, the alveoli and their capillaries are lined by cells that create a nearly watertight barrier. So long as those barriers remain intact, little fluid can pass from capillaries to alveoli. Chemicals can disrupt those barriers, however, and make the alveoli leaky or permeable. Pulmonary edema that forms when alveoli and capillaries become permeable is known as noncardio-genic or permeability pulmonary edema.

Under normal conditions, a small amount of fluid passes from the capillaries into the alveoli. To maintain the alveoli as dry as possible, the alveolar lining cells pump that fluid out of the alveoli and back into the blood vessels. This pumping of fluid, which requires cellular energy, is a second mechanism by which the lung prevents pulmonary edema. Chemicals that disrupt cellular energy production (such as cyanide or hydrogen sulfide) interfere with this mechanism and decrease the ability of alveolar cells to pump fluid and keep the alveoli dry. Exposure to such chemicals can, therefore, produce pulmonary edema.

A third protective mechanism is provided by *surfactant,* a fatty substance secreted by type II alveolar cells. Surfactant reduces the *surface tension* of the alveoli, a process that helps to keep the alveoli from collapsing. If the alveolar surface tension increases, fluid is drawn from capillaries into the alveoli, and pulmonary edema forms. Disruption of surfactant, therefore, leads to increased alveolar surface tension and pulmonary edema.

Surfactant can be disturbed by exposure to many reactive chemicals. It can be dissolved or precipitated by acids and alkali. Other chemicals can damage the cells that produce surfactant. Damage to those cells results in decreased surfactant production and abnormal alveolar surface tension. These disturbances can evolve slowly and result in delayed pulmonary edema developing 12 to 24 hours after chemical exposure.

Unlike cardiogenic pulmonary edema that results from heart failure, permeability pulmonary edema is not caused by disturbed heart work or blood pressure. On the basis of clinical examination, however, it is not possible to distinguish patients with permeability pulmonary edema from those with congestive heart failure. Victims suffer respiratory distress, cyanosis, rapid pulse, and diaphoresis. Rales and crackles can be heard in the lungs and there may be frothy or bloody sputum.

It is important to remember that pulmonary edema may not develop for hours or days after inhalation exposure to chemicals. At the time of a victim's initial assessment, it is impossible to assure him or her that edema will not develop. For this reason, all inhalation exposure victims must be carefully evaluated and regularly reassessed to assure that pulmonary edema is promptly recognized (Figure 15–7).

SUMMARY

Inhalation of hazardous chemicals can cause a variety of toxic effects on the lungs and airways. In thinking about those effects, it is useful to divide the lung into three anatomic sections: the conducting airways, bronchiolar airways, and alveoli.

Chemicals that are water soluble tend to affect the larger airways, whereas

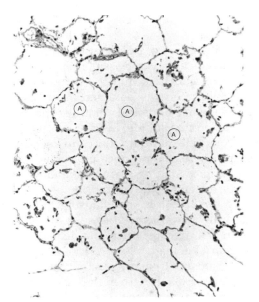

Figure 15–7a Light microscopic picture of normal alveoli. Note that the individual alveoli are empty except for occasional debris and artifact. (Courtesy of G. J. Walker Smith, M.D., Yale University School of Medicine, New Haven, Conn.)

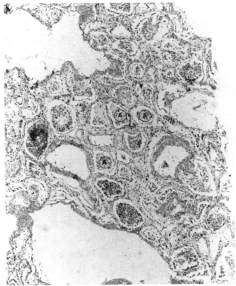

Figure 15–7b Light microscopic picture of alveoli filled by permeability pulmonary edema. The dark staining material within the alveoli represents protein-rich edema fluid. Of note is the thickening of the alveolar membrane (A = alveoli). (Courtesy of G. J. Walker Smith, M.D., Yale University School of Medicine, New Haven, Conn.)

water-insoluble chemicals are more likely to affect the alveoli. Other factors that determine the kinds of pulmonary injury caused by toxic inhalation include the reactivity of the chemical, its concentration, the duration of exposure, and the condition of the victim at the time of inhalation.

The effects of toxic inhalation can be delayed. It is important, therefore, that a careful assessment of the lungs be carried out followed by regular reassessments. An initially normal examination can occur despite serious injury in a victim. Some victims develop life-threatening pulmonary edema or asthma after a delay of 6 to 12 hours or more.

REFERENCES

AKINO, T., and K. OHNO, ''Phospholipids of the Lung in Normal, Toxic and Diseased States,'' *CRC Crit. Rev. Toxicol.*, 9 (1981), 201–74.

ALARIE, Y., "Sensory Irritation of the Upper Airways by Airborne Chemicals," *Toxicol. Appl. Pharmacol.*, 24 (1973), 279–97.

ALBERT, R. K., S. LAKSHMINARAYAN, J. HILDEBRANDT, et al., "Increased Surface Tension Favors Pulmonary Edema Formation in Anesthetized Dogs' Lungs," *J. Clin. Invest.*, 63 (1979), 1015–18.

BASSET, F., V. J. FERRANS, P. SOLER, et al., "Intraluminal Fibrosis in Interstitial Lung Disorders," *Am. J. Pathol.*, 122 (1986), 443–61.

BERNARD, G. R., and K. L. BRIGHAM, "Pulmonary Edema: Pathophysiologic Mechanisms and New Approaches to Therapy," *Chest*, 89 (1986), 594–600.

DEMLING, R. H., "Role of Prostaglandins in Acute Pulmonary Microvascular Injury," *Ann. N.Y. Acad. Sci.*, 384 (1982), 517–34.

DIXON, M., and D. M. NEEDHAM, "Biochemical Research on Chemical Warfare Agents," *Nature*, 158 (1946), 432–38.

EVANS, M. J., "Oxidant Gases," *Environ. Health. Perspect.*, 55 (1984), 85–95.

FAIRCHILD, E. J., and S. L. GRAHAM, "Thyroid Influence on the Toxicity of Respiratory Irritant Gases, Ozone and Nitrogen Dioxide," *J. Pharmacol. Exp. Ther.*, 139 (1963), 177–84.

GROPPER, M. A., and M. A. MATTHAY, "Resolution of Pulmonary Edema," *Hospital Physician*, 1988 (1988), 70–74.

HAAGSMAN, H. P., and L. M. G. VAN GOLDE, "Lung Surfactant and Pulmonary Toxicology," *Lung*, 163 (1985), 275–303.

HOLLINGER, M. A., *Respiratory Pharmacology and Toxicology*. Philadelphia: W. B. Saunders Company, 1985.

KILBURN, K. H., "Particles Causing Lung Disease," *Environ. Health Perspect.*, 55 (1984), 97–109.

MANNY, J., N. MANNY, S. LELCUK, et al., "Pulmonary and Systemic Consequences of Localized Acid Aspiration," *Surg. Gynecol. Obstet.*, 162 (1986), 259–66.

MENZEL, D. B., and M. O. AMDUR, "Toxic Responses of the Respiratory System," in *Casarett and Doull's Toxicology: The Basic Science of Poisons*, pp. 330–57, eds. C. D. Klaassen, M. O. Amdur, and J. Doull. New York: Macmillan Publishing Co., Inc., 1986.

MEYRICK, B. O., "Pathology of Pulmonary Edema," *Semin. Respir. Med.*, 4 (1983), 267–73.

SCHWARTZ, D. A., "Acute Inhalation Injury," *Occup. Med. State Art Rev.*, 2 (1987), 297–317.

SMITH, L. L., G. M. COHEN, and W. N. ALDRIDGE, "Morphological and Biochemical Correlates of Chemical Induced Injury in the Lung," *Arch Toxicol.*, 58 (1986), 214–18.

STAUB, N. C., "Pulmonary Edema due to Increased Microvascular Permeability to Fluid and Protein," *Circ. Res.*, 43 (1978), 143–51.

SUMMER, W., and E. HAPONIK, "Inhalation of Irritant Gases," *Clin. Chest Med.,* 2 (1981), 273–87.

TRANBAUGH, R. F., and F. R. LEWIS, "Mechanisms and Etiologic Factors of Pulmonary Edema," *Surg. Gynecol. Obstet.,* 158 (1984), 193–206.

WEST, J. B., *Respiratory Physiology.* Baltimore, Md.: Williams & Wilkins, 1974.

ACUTE CHEMICAL INJURIES OF THE EYE

CHAPTER 16

GOAL: On completion of this chapter the student will have an understanding of the basic mechanisms by which chemicals cause eye injuries, will understand why exposure to alkali can cause the severest eye injuries, and will understand the basic principles of emergency care for chemical eye burns.

OBJECTIVES:

Specifically, the student will be able to

- Define coagulation, liquefaction, and ischemic necroses
- Explain why exposures to alkali can cause severer eye injury than exposures to acids
- Describe the types of eye injuries likely to be caused by exposure to solvents, detergents and surfactants, and lacrimators
- Explain why all chemical eye burns should be managed as though severe injury had occurred

OVERVIEW

This chapter focuses on the toxic effects of hazardous chemicals on the eyes. First, the anatomy and architecture of the eyes will be reviewed as related to toxic exposures. Next, the similarities and differences in the ways that acids and alkali cause ocular damage will be examined. Finally, the ocular effects of some other types of chemicals will be discussed.

Eye injuries frequently result from accidental exposure to hazardous chemicals. It is estimated that chemical injuries represent 10 percent of eye trauma in industrial settings. Because the eyes are delicate and vulnerable, injuries to them must be regarded as potential causes of blindness. Fortunately, only a minority of toxic eye injuries are severe enough to cause loss of sight.

Severe eye injuries are most often due to the effects of acids and alkali, but other chemicals including amines, vesicants, and alkylating agents can cause devastating damage. In most cases, the eyes are directly exposed to splashed liquids, concentrated vapors, or particles of chemical dust. Less often, acute chemical-induced visual changes are due to the systemic effects of intoxication. Methanol poisoning is one example of a systemic intoxication frequently associated with visual disturbances and blindness. Emergency response personnel can suffer eye injuries following exposure to smoke, chemical splashes, splashed water that has been contaminated by chemicals, or exposure to gases, dusts, and fumes.

ANATOMIC CONSIDERATIONS

The human eye is a spheroidal body about 1 inch in diameter. It consists of anterior and posterior portions that have different functions and different vulnerabilities to chemical injuries. The anterior portion of the eye is in front of (or external to) the lens. As seen in Figure 16–1, it includes the cornea, the conjunctiva, the iris, the anterior chamber (filled with aqueous humor), and the eyelids. These ocular structures primarily serve to admit and focus light entering the eye. The anterior portion is exposed directly to the environment and can be injured by chemical contact owing to liquid splash or vapor contact.

The *sclera* is a tough, fibrous membrane that forms the outer surface of the eyeball including the white of the eye. It is continuous with the *cornea*, which is clear and transparent. The transparent cornea allows light to enter the eye. The sclera and cornea are covered by a thin membrane, the *conjunctiva*, which also lines the underside of the eyelids.

The cornea is made up of two thin layers of cells that coat a thicker, fibrous material called the *corneal stroma*. The outer layer of cells helps to keep chemicals and other foreign material from penetrating into the stroma and deeper structures of the eye. Chemical-induced changes to the corneal stroma and its outer layer of cells can lead to blindness by causing the cornea to become opacified. The cornea must remain transparent to be functional.

The surface of a healthy eye is kept moist by tears that are secreted by the *lacrimal glands*. Water-soluble chemicals (such as most acids and alkali) are attracted to and dissolve in the surface water that coats the eye. Vapors of reactive chemicals can cause severe and rapidly evolving injuries.

The *anterior chamber* is the space between the back of the cornea and the front of the lens. It is filled by a fluid called *aqueous humor*. Chemicals that are able to penetrate the cornea enter the anterior chamber and then diffuse throughout the eye. The *iris* is the colored part of the eye. The *pupil* is an adjust-

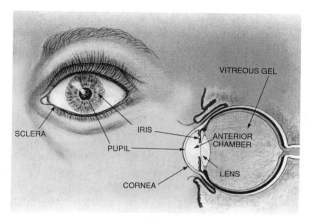

Figure 16–1a The anatomy of the anterior portion of the eye. (Slide no. 10, "Introduction to Ophthalmology," reprinted with permission, The American Academy of Ophthalmology.)

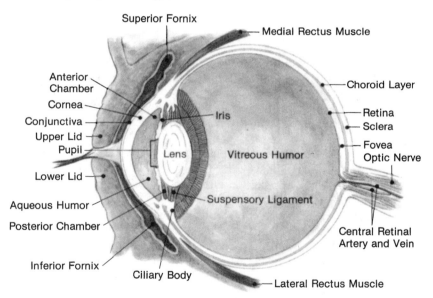

Figure 16–1b Anatomy of the eye as seen on cross-section.

able opening in the iris that becomes larger or smaller and controls the amount of light entering the eye. Irritating chemicals that penetrate into the anterior chamber can cause inflammation and damage to the iris.

The posterior portion of the eye includes the retina, optic nerve, and vitreous humor-filled posterior chamber. This part of the eye acts as a receiver that converts light into the neurological activity of vision. The posterior portion lies deep within the bony orbit. It is shielded from direct chemical exposure by the orbit and skull bones, periorbital soft tissues, and anterior portion of the eye. Only rarely do the posterior eye structures come into direct contact with harmful industrial chemicals. When that happens, it is usually after massive injury to the anterior portion of the eye.

EFFECTS OF ACIDS AND ALKALI

Acids and alkali are the chemicals that most often cause serious eye injury. Severe damage and blindness can result from exposure to concentrated solutions of either. In general, alkali are more damaging than acids. This is primarily because of the greater ability of alkali to penetrate the cornea and enter into the deep areas of the eye. Concentrated acid solutions, however, are as devastating to the eye as are strong alkali.

Penetration by Acids and Alkali

When strong acids contact the eye, either as a splash of liquid or as concentrated vapor, an immediate reaction causes proteins to precipitate and form a clotlike coagulum that covers the cornea with an opaque, white membrane. This process, which is often associated with cell death, is known as *coagulation necrosis*. The coagulum itself can absorb and buffer acid. As a result, that coagulum becomes a barrier that protects the eye by blocking deeper penetration of the acid. The coagulum is usually thin and superficial; clear, living cornea is often underneath.

Acids must be strong to penetrate beneath the coagulum. For example, an acid cannot penetrate deeply into a normal eye unless its pH is less than 2. The destructive effects of an acid at a pH less than 2, however, are about as great as those caused by strong alkali.

Alkali penetrate the eye's outer membranes more easily than acids. This is related to the ability of alkali to dissolve fats and fatlike substances. Alkali remove fatty substances called *lipids* from the cell membranes. Affected cells die, and their membranes fall apart. The contents of the cells and the remains of their membranes are turned into a slimy, liquified material. This process is known as *liquefaction necrosis*. Unlike acid-induced coagulation necrosis, alkali-induced liquefaction necrosis does not provide any barrier to deep penetration by alkali. In fact, liquefaction necrosis contributes to rapid penetration by alkali because the alkali diffuse readily through the liquified cellular material.

After contact with strong alkali, cells covering the cornea are disrupted and damaged, and no longer serve as a barrier to penetration. In some cases, penetration of alkali into the anterior chamber is almost immediate. For example, ammonia, a potent alkali, was found in the aqueous humor within 5 seconds after it was applied experimentally to the cornea of laboratory animals. After only 20 seconds, the pH of the anterior chamber had begun to rise. Because alkali can generally penetrate more rapidly and deeper than acids, a much deeper injury usually occurs.

The cellular lining of the cornea is an important barrier to penetration of chemicals, especially acids. If the lining is disrupted as a result of corneal abrasions or puncture wounds, acids are able to penetrate as rapidly and deeply as alkali. In that event, acids and alkali of equal strength cause equal damage to the eye. This points to the important role of the cornea as protection against chemical exposure injuries.

Effects on Corneal Stroma

The corneal stroma consist mainly of connective tissue fibers called *collagen* and complex sugars called *mucopoly saccharides* that coat the collagen fibers. Collagen represents about 80 percent of the corneal stroma, and complex sugars account for nearly all the rest. Protein- and salt-rich tissue water flows around and between the fibers of collagen.

Strong acids and strong alkali have different effects on the corneal stroma. Acids cause proteins to precipitate, a process that can result in corneal opacification. Acids also damage the cells that line the cornea and lead to swelling and edema of the stroma. In general, however, acids do not affect the collagen fibers or the mucopolysaccharides coating them. Moreover, the opacification caused by acids is usually superficial, involving only the formation of a protein coagulum on the cornea's outer surface. Acids only rarely opacify the corneal stroma.

By contrast, alkali dissolve and remove the complex sugars that normally coat and protect corneal collagen fibers. Naked collagen fibers quickly become swollen and edematous. Alkali can also cause proteins in the corneal stroma to precipitate. The combined effects of collagen fiber swelling, protein precipitation, and edema of the stroma can lead to severe corneal opacification and blindness. Moreover, removal of the complex sugar coating from collagen fibers makes them vulnerable to delayed injury. Such injuries include corneal ulcers that can perforate and cause loss of the eye.

In most cases, the effects of alkali on the corneal stroma are much greater than those caused by acids.

Effects on the Ocular Vasculature

Arteries and veins are easily damaged when they come into contact with strong acids or alkali. Such contact causes clots or *thromboses* to form and block the affected blood vessels. Cells that depended on the thrombosed vessels to supply oxygen may die from lack of oxygen, a process called *ischemic necrosis*.

When strong acids or alkali splash into the eye, the blood vessels that feed the cornea can be burned and thrombosed. Ischemic necrosis of the cornea then often results. Injuries of this kind are among the worst that the eye can suffer and usually lead to blindness or loss of the eye.

Effects on the Anterior Chamber

Strong acids and alkali can penetrate the cornea and enter the anterior chamber. Once in the aqueous humor, the chemicals can diffuse throughout the eye to cause damage to deeper structures. The iris is particularly vulnerable to chemical injury.

It is possible to monitor the penetration of acids and alkali into the eye experimentally by measuring the pH of the anterior chamber. For example, the pH effects caused by corneal application of an alkali, sodium hydroxide, is shown in Figure 16–2. The rapid increase of anterior chamber pH can be seen. The pH remained dangerously elevated for hours, even when the eye was continuously washed with water.

Acid exposure causes less severe changes of the anterior chamber pH than exposures to alkali. The pH abnormalities develop more slowly after exposure and remain abnormal for a shorter period of time. Washing an acid exposed with water can quickly return the pH to normal.

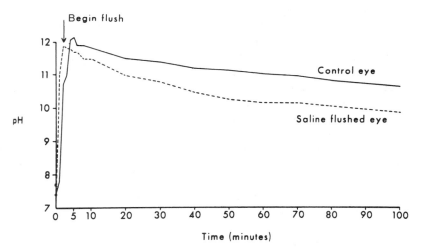

Figure 16–2 Effects of pH on anterior chamber of cornea following application of sodium hydroxide, a powerful alkali. Control eye received no wash, whereas the saline-flushed eye was irrigated continuously after application of alkali. (From Paterson, C. A., R. R. Pfister, and R. A. Levinson, "Aqueous Humor pH Changes after Experimental Alkali Burns," *Am. J. Ophthalmol.*, 79 [1975], 3; published with permission from The American Journal of Ophthalmology. Copyright by The Ophthalmic Publishing Company.)

It is important to bring the anterior chamber pH back to normal as soon as possible after acid or alkali exposure. This helps to limit the damage caused by the exposure. As discussed subsequently, it is often necessary to provide continuous water or saline irrigation of the eyes for hours to save the sight of exposure victims.

Clinical Effects of Exposure

It is not possible to judge the severity of a chemical eye burn until 48 hours or more after exposure. In some cases, the initial appearance of the injured eye suggests much greater damage than has actually occurred. In others, an apparently mild exposure leads to total blindness or loss of the eye.

Acid eye burns, for example, can appear to cause immediate opacification and blindness because of the protein coagulum formed by acid-induced coagulation necrosis. This suggests severe injury. In fact, however, the underlying cornea may be normal and healthy, and no permanent loss of vision may have occurred. By contrast, opacification after alkali exposure can be delayed. At first the eye can seem almost normal, yet the burn may be so severe that blindness develops or the eye is lost.

The appearance of eyes shortly after alkali burns of various severity is presented in Figure 16–3. The grading of the severity of eye burns in that figure is intended only as a general guide. At first, little discriminates between the presentation of a mild versus a moderate to severe burn. With proper care, however the mild burn will heal without visual loss, whereas the moderate to severe burn will probably cause reduced vision.

The progressive damage that can occur after eye exposure to strong alkali and other chemicals is demonstrated in Figure 16–4. This figure shows the same eye immediately after exposure and months later after corneal scarring has caused opacification and blindness. It is not possible to determine the severity of a chemical eye injury immediately following exposure. Emergency responders must manage all chemical eye exposures as severe injuries.

Blindness owing to corneal opacification is one of the long-term effects of acid and alkali exposures. Ulceration and perforation leading to loss of the eye also occurs after severe exposures, especially those causing ischemic necrosis of the cornea. In some cases, the healing of chemical burns of the conjunctiva causes scarring that interferes with eyelid movement and closure, a condition called *symblepharon*.

Management of Exposure Victims

Prompt and continuous irrigation with water or saline is the single most important aspect of caring for chemically exposed eyes. As described in chapter 13, irrigation of the eye can be carried out by several different methods. As a general

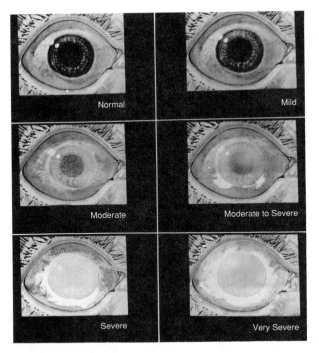

Figure 16–3 Classification of alkali-burned eyes. *Normal eye; mild:* corneal epithelial erosion, faint anterior haziness, no ischemic necrosis; *moderate:* moderate corneal opacity, little ischemic necrosis; *moderate to severe:* corneal opacity, blurring iris, ischemic necrosis of less than one-third of conjunctiva; *severe:* blurring of pupils' outline, ischemia of one-third to two-thirds of conjunctiva, cornea often opaque; *very severe:* pupil not visible, ischemia of greater than two-thirds of conjunctiva, completely opaque cornea. (Pfister, Roswell R., ''Chemical Injuries of the Eye,'' *South. Med. J.*, 75 [1982], 418; reprinted with permission.)

rule, irrigation must be carried out for at least 15 minutes after most exposures and at least 20 minutes after exposure to alkali. It is also important that rescuers make efforts to assure that no foreign bodies or solid particles of chemicals are left in the eye or under the eyelids.

If an eye exposure victim is wearing contact lenses, it is generally best to remove those lenses to irrigate the eye. It may be necessary to use a lens removal suction bulb. Lens removal should be performed carefully to avoid causing further injury to the cornea. If a contact lens cannot be easily removed, however, slide it away from the iris onto the sclera and continue washing the eye.

Rescuers must also remember that the eye is fragile after alkali burns. Rough handling or excessive pressure can cause its surface to be torn and perfo-

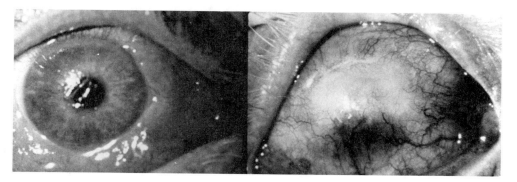

Figure 16–4 Progressive damage to the eye occurs particularly after exposure to strong alkali. It is important that rescuers not judge the severity of an eye exposure until at least 48 hours after injury. *Left:* Alkali-injured eye within hours of exposure. The severity of injury cannot be judged. *Right:* Severe, chronic changes developed over the next several months; pupil is not visible, cornea is totally opacified, and vision has been completely lost (Slide no. 7, ''Eye Trauma and Emergencies,'' reprinted with permission, American Academy of Ophthalmology.)

rate. To protect the eye, it should be touched and handled as little as possible while the victim is transported to a definitive medical care facility.

SOLVENTS

Solvents are pH-neutral chemicals that are used industrially for their ability to dissolve other substances. Examples include benzene, toluene, alcohols such as ethanol and isopropanol, and hydrocarbons such as gasoline. Many solvents can dissolve and remove fat from living tissues. These solvents are known as *defatting agents.*

Fats are removed from cells on the corneal surface when solvents are splashed into the eye. Unlike alkali, which dissolve fats and cause liquefaction necrosis, solvents do not generally destroy cells. The corneal lining cells may be disturbed, however, and the cornea may become swollen by edema. Victims may experience blurred or abnormal vision for several days.

The effects of solvents on the eye are almost never serious. Severe stinging pain can occur, and the cornea may appear dull instead of shiny. Healing usually occurs within several days, however. Long-term effects rarely result.

The management of these exposure victims involves gentle eye irrigation. After ocular exposure to pure solvents, continuous eye washing for several minutes may be enough. It is better to be cautious and safe, however, by irrigating for at least 15 minutes. The same eye irrigation techniques described earlier for acids and alkali should be used.

DETERGENTS AND SURFACTANTS

Many chemicals are used industrially because they lower the surface tension of water and help to dissolve fatty substances. Such chemicals are known as detergents, emulsifiers, wetting agents, antifoaming agents and solubilizers.

Many of these compounds are irritating to the eyes. They cause intense stinging pain and inflammation of the conjunctiva after eye contact. The eye pain caused by soap or shampoo is an example of mild injury caused by detergents and surfactants. More powerful compounds can cause protein precipitation similar to that caused by exposure to acids. Others cause damage like that owing to strong alkali, including corneal opacification and blindness.

Following exposure, the cornea may appear dulled instead of shiny. Inflammation of the conjunctiva gives the eye a blood-shot appearance. The cornea is often swollen with edema.

The management of exposure victims primarily involves irrigation of the eyes for at least 15 minutes as described above.

LACRIMATORS

Lacrimators are chemicals that are reactive and usually water soluble. Exposure to low concentrations of chemical vapors causes profuse tear formation. In low concentrations, lacrimators act as tear gases. Exposure to high vapor concentrations or liquid splashes of these chemicals, conversely, can cause massive destruction. Under those conditions, these chemicals act as vesicants. Examples include acrolein, mace, ethyl benzene, and fresh onions.

Exposure causes immediate stinging pain and tearing. After low-dose exposure, injury is usually minor and limited. As the dose increases, the cornea and conjunctiva become inflamed. At high doses, injury can cause opacification of the cornea and blindness. The periorbital soft tissues, including the eyelids, can also be burned.

The management of these exposure victims, like those previously described, involves continuous irrigation of the eyes for at least 15 minutes. Use the same eye irrigation techniques that were described earlier. Intense tearing may continue for hours even after adequate irrigation. When medically approved, application of a topical anesthetic such as proparacaine hydrochloride (one or two drops of a 0.5 percent solution in each eye) can relieve symptomatic complaints.

DELAYED CORNEAL INJURIES

Some chemicals cause delayed corneal effects following exposure. Many of these are gases that dissolve in the corneal surface water and then injure the eye. Generally, such chemicals cause tissue disturbances that result in delayed cell death. Most are alkylating agents (such as formaldehyde and ethylene oxide) or enzyme poisons (such as hydrogen sulfide).

Typically, exposure to these chemicals causes no symptoms or complaints for several hours or more. Then victims begin to suffer burning irritation, blurred vision, "halos" around lights, and discomfort when looking at bright lights. The cornea may appear dulled and without luster.

Effects can last for several days. In rare situations, eye damage can be severe and lead to corneal ulcers and eye loss.

The management of these victims should include eye wash as described earlier for at least 15 minutes even though exposure may have occurred hours before. Cool compresses to the eyes may be soothing. The use of a drop of olive oil in affected eyes can provide symptomatic relief.

SUMMARY

Because the eye is so delicate an organ, it is readily injured by chemicals of many sorts. Any chemical injury poses a threat of blindness. The most dangerous exposures are caused by acids and alkali. Many other compounds can disturb vision.

The eye's natural protective mechanisms against chemical injuries include the cornea and its external cell layer, which block the penetration of toxic substances. Chemicals that disturb that penetration barrier, especially alkali, can penetrate rapidly and cause deep injury. Disturbances of the cornea, such as abrasions, increase the speed and severity of chemical exposure injuries.

Management of eye exposure victims depends primarily on removal of the offending chemical by copious washing. At least 15 minutes of continuous irrigation is necessary for most chemicals. Following exposure to alkali, irrigation should be carried out for at least 20 minutes and, if possible, continuous washing should take place until the patient is transported to a definitive medical care facility.

REFERENCES

Bronstein, A. C., and P. L. Currance, *Emergency Care for Hazardous Materials Exposure.* St. Louis: The C. V. Mosby Company, 1988.

Chiang, T. S., L. R. Moorman, and R. P. Thomas, "Ocular Hypertensive Response Following Acid and Alkali Burns in Rabbits," *Invest. Ophthalmol. Vis. Sci.* 10 (1971), 270–73.

DIXON, M., and D. M. NEEDHAM, "Biochemical Research on Chemical Warfare Agents," *Nature* 158 (1946), 432–38.

FLYNN, W. J., T. F. MAUGER, and R. M. HILL, "Corneal Burns: A Quantitative Comparison of Acid and Base," *Acta. Ophthalmol.*, 62 (1984), 542–48.

FRIEDENWALD, J. S., W. F. HUGHES, and H. HERRMANN, "Acid-Base Tolerance of the Cornea," *Arch. Ophthalmol.*, 31 (1944), 279–83.

GONNERING, R., H. F. EDELHAUSER, D. L. VAN HORN, et al., "pH Tolerance of Rabbit and Human Corneal Endothelium," *Invest. Ophthalmol. Vis. Sci.*, 18 (1979), 373–90.

GRANT, W. M., *Toxicology of the Eye.* Springfield, Ill.: Charles C Thomas, 1986.

HUGHES, W. F., "Alkali Burns of the Eye: I. Review of the Literature and Summary of Present Knowledge," *Arch. Ophthalmol.*, 35 (1946), 423–49.

HUGHES, W. F., "Alkali Burns of the Eye: II. Clinical and Pathologic Course," *Arch. Ophthalmol.*, 36 (1946), 189–214.

LEMP, M. A., "Cornea and Sclera," *Arch. Ophthalmol.*, 92 (1974), 158–70.

MAUGER, T. F., and R. M. HILL, "Epithelial Healing: Quantitative Monitoring of the Cornea Following Alkali Burn," *Acta Ophthalmol.*, 63 (1985), 264–67.

MCLAUGHLIN, R. S., "Chemical Burns of the Human Cornea," *Am. J. Ophthalmol.*, 29 (1946), 1355–62.

NELSON, J. D., and L. A. KOPIETZ, "Chemical Injuries to the Eyes: Emergency, Intermediate, and Long-Term Care," *Postgrad. Med. J.*, 81 (1987), 62–75.

PATERSON, C. A., and R. R. PFISTER, "Prostaglandin-like Activity in the Aqueous Humor Following Alkali Burns," *Invest. Ophthalmol. Vis. Sci.*, 14 (1975), 177–83.

PATERSON, C. A., R. R. PFISTER, and R. A. LEVINSON, "Aqueous Humor pH Changes after Experimental Alkali Burns," *Am. J. Ophthalmol.*, 79 (1975), 414–19.

PFISTER, R. R., "Chemical Injuries of the Eye," *Ophthalmology,* 90 (1983), 1246–53.

POTTS, A. M., "Toxic Responses of the Eye," in *Casarett and Doull's Toxicology: The Basic Science of Poisons.* pp. 478–517, eds. C. D. Klaassen, M. O. Amdur, and J. Doull. New York: Macmillan Publishing Co., Inc., 1986.

RALPH, R. A., and H. H. SLANSKY, "Therapy of Chemical Burns," in *Practical Management of Ocular Injuries*, pp. 171–91, ed. S. A. Boruchoff. Boston: Little, Brown & Company, 1974.

ROSEMAN, M. J., and R. M. HILL, "Aerobic Responses of the Cornea to Isopropyl Alcohol, Measured in Vivo," *Acta Ophthalmol.*, 65 (1987), 306–12.

WRIGHT, P. "Chemically Injured Eye," *Trans. Ophthalmol. Soc. U.K.*, 102 (1982), 85–87.

ACUTE CHEMICAL INJURIES OF THE SKIN

CHAPTER 17

GOAL: On completion of this chapter the student will understand the mechanisms by which chemicals can injure the skin, will understand the factors that determine the severity of such skin injuries, and will understand the basic principles of emergency skin care for chemical burns.

OBJECTIVES:

Specifically, the student will be able to

- Name six mechanisms by which chemicals can cause skin injury
- Define contact dermatitis, vesiculation, and corrosion
- List four factors that determine the severity of chemical skin injury
- Explain the essential first step in the management of chemical exposures of the skin
- Name some of the complications associated with severe chemical skin burns
- Describe special concerns for managing victims of skin exposure to hydrofluoric acid, phosphorus, alkali metals (such as sodium and lithium), and phenol

OVERVIEW

This chapter is concerned with those skin injuries that can result from acute exposure to toxic chemicals. First, some aspects of skin anatomy are reviewed that relate to toxic exposures. Next, some types of skin injury caused by hazardous chemicals and the factors that determine their severity are considered. Finally, several toxic chemicals that pose unique problems and require unusual care are discussed.

The skin is the organ that establishes our physical boundary with the outside world. It is one of the largest body organs, representing about 10 percent of total body weight. Because of its constant exposure to foreign materials, the skin is the organ most frequently injured by toxic chemicals. Nearly half of all work-related toxic exposures and accidents cause skin disorders. In addition, many skin injuries result from chemical exposures at home and during nonoccupational accidents.

The most common chemical-induced skin diseases are allergic reactions and contact dermatitis. It is estimated that these patients account for as much as 40 percent of all occupational disease cases. Most are due to chronic or repeated exposures to hazardous substances. A smaller group, about 10 percent of all occupational disease patients, suffer skin disease caused by acute, accidental skin contaminations and chemical skin burns. Although smaller in number, the patients in this acute skin exposure group include the most serious toxic skin injuries and chemical burns.

ANATOMIC CONSIDERATIONS

The skin consists of two principal layers: *epidermis*, the outer layer, and *dermis*, the deeper layer (Figure 17–1). The epidermis consists primarily of live and metabolically active cells. Overlying the epidermis is a superficial membrane of dead, dried cells called the *corneum stratum* (Figure 17–2).

The corneum stratum acts as a protective barrier that prevents foreign materials from making contact with the living cells of the epidermis. Toxic chemicals must penetrate that barrier before they can cause harm. Most water-soluble chemicals penetrate the corneum stratum slowly and, therefore, have limited ability to cause skin injury. A few, such as alkali, dissolve the barrier and produce rapid, severe damage.

When the corneum stratum is absent or disrupted, chemical exposure leads to severer and more rapid skin damage. No corneum stratum is under the fingernails and toenails, for example, and the nail beds are therefore vulnerable to chemical injuries. Acids, particularly hydrofluoric acid, cause severe burns of the nail beds. These burns can lead to loss of fingers and toes. Skin abrasions and lacerations disrupt the corneum stratum. For this reason, traumatized skin is more vulnerable to toxic exposures than normal skin.

The epidermis contains only a few cells, blood vessels, nerve endings, fat deposits, and skin appendages such as hair follicles, sweat glands, and other types of skin glands. Blood vessels are in the dermis but not in the epidermis. Injuries to the epidermis do not bleed. If a skin injury does bleed, it must have involved the dermis.

Chemicals must penetrate through the epidermis and into the blood ves-

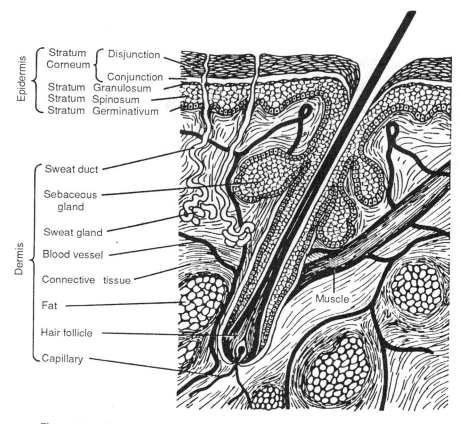

Figure 17–1 The cross-sectional anatomy of the skin. (Reprinted by permission of Macmillan Publishing Company from *Casarett and Doull's Toxicology, The Basic Science of Poisons, 3rd ed.*, p. 414, by Klaassen, C. D., Ph.D., Amdur, M., and Doull, M.D., Ph.D. Copyright ©1986 Macmillan Publishing Company, a division of Macmillan, Inc.)

sels of the dermis to be absorbed and cause systemic poisoning. Skin absorption of chemicals is known as *percutaneous absorption*. The effects of chemicals that undergo percutaneous absorption will be considered later in chapter 18.

MECHANISMS OF SKIN INJURY BY CHEMICALS

Toxic skin damage can be caused by several different mechanisms. In some cases, only a single mechanism is active. In other cases, however, injury results from the combined effects of two or more mechanisms that each causes harm. Six different mechanisms of injury are as follows:

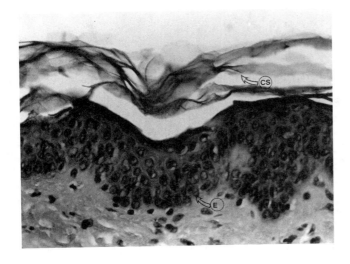

Figure 17–2 Light microscopic picture of the skin showing the epidermis (E) and the corneum stratum (CS). (Courtesy of B. J. Longley, Jr., M.D., Yale University School of Medicine, New Haven, Conn.)

1. Thermal injuries: cold

2. Thermal injuries: heat

3. Mechanical injuries

4. Ischemic necrosis

5. Irritation

6. Chemical burns and corrosion

Thermal Injuries: Cold

Many common chemicals that exist as gases under normal conditions are stored as liquids under increased pressure. Chlorine and ammonia are two examples of chemicals that are routinely stored in this way. When liquefied chemical gases escape from their high-pressure containers, they rapidly expand and absorb heat. Skin or other living tissues that are exposed to gas escaping from high pressure storage will suffer freeze injury and frostbite.

Thermal Injuries: Heat

More than 65 percent of all hazardous materials incidents are due to spills and leaks of flammable liquids. At such incidents, great risk of fires and thermal burns exists. Emergency responders at incidents involving these chemicals must be prepared to care for the victims of thermal burns.

Thermal burns are also a risk at chemical plants when manufacturing processes are carried out at high temperatures. Explosions or spills of hot chemicals can lead to thermal burns.

In addition, some chemicals produce heat by reacting with body tissues. For example, sulfuric acid reacts with water to yield large amounts of heat. If sulfuric acid is spilt on the skin, it reacts with tissue water and produces enough heat to cause thermal burns of the skin and underlying tissues. Heat is also produced when acids or alkali are *neutralized,* that is, when acids are added to alkali, or alkali are added to acids. The heat produced by neutralization reactions can cause thermal burns. For that reason, acids and alkali should not be neutralized if they are spilt on the skin.

Mechanical Injuries

Some chemicals cause injury by producing violent mechanical damage to exposed cells. An example is the dehydrating effect of concentrated acids such as sulfuric and hydrochloric. When those acids contact living tissues, they exert powerful forces that draw water out of cells. Affected cells suffer violent mechanical dehydration, or *desiccation,* and die.

Ischemic Necrosis

Arteries and veins are easily damaged when they come into contact with strong acids, alkali, and some other corrosive chemicals. Such contact causes clots or *thromboses* to form and block the affected blood vessels. Cells that depended on the thrombosed vessels to supply oxygen may die from lack of oxygen, a process called *ischemic necrosis.* This process was described in chapter 16.

Corrosive chemicals that penetrate the epidermis and enter the dermis are likely to cause injury to dermal blood vessels. Ischemic necrosis can then result, adding to the tissue damage caused by the corrosives. Ischemic necrosis is unlikely to occur in this way unless extensive corrosive tissue damage has occurred. Therefore, ischemic necrosis is of less importance in producing toxic skin injuries than toxic eye injuries.

Irritation

Cutaneous irritation occurs when chemical skin contact causes inflammation of the skin not resulting from an allergic reaction. The inflammatory skin reaction caused by a skin irritant is called *contact dermatitis.*

Acute irritation develops after a single exposure to a chemical. Chronic or cumulative irritation develops after chronic or repeated exposures. Acute irritants are generally more potent or more concentrated than those that cause cumulative irritation. Some are capable of causing severe skin burns following high-dose or prolonged exposures. Chemicals that can cause acute irritation and contact dermatitis include acids, alkali, vesicants, and solvents.

Irritation causes the skin to become reddened and swollen. In severer cases, blisters, or *vesiculation,* and scaling of the skin may also occur. Distinctive skin changes are usually not immediately present. Following exposure, irritation and dermatitis can develop over hours or days. Acute contact dermatitis is usually self-limited and reversible. Only rarely does contact dermatitis develop into a chronic condition or cause scar formation or other skin abnormalities.

Chemical Burns and Corrosion

Some chemicals are very destructive and cause irreversible damage to the tissues they contact. Those chemicals are often referred to as *corrosives,* and their effect on the tissues is called *corrosion.* Corrosion causes the skin to dissolve or disintegrate, and results in loss of cell and tissue structures. Skin contact with corrosives leads to cell death, ulcerations, and loss of skin. Severe corrosive injuries are often called *chemical burns.*

The commonest causes of chemical burns are acids and alkali. Important differences exist between the tissue effects of acids and alkali. As described in chapter 9, acids cause *coagulation necrosis,* a process that leads to the precipitation of protein as a clotlike coagulum. The protein coagulum absorbs and buffers acid and prevents deep penetration. As a result, acid burns tend to be superficial injuries. Acid skin burns usually appear dry and crusted. The color of the burn crust depends on the specific acid causing the burn.

Alkali cause the fatty substances of cell membranes to dissolve and causes those cells to disintegrate, a process called *liquefaction necrosis.* Unlike coagulation necrosis, alkali-induced liquefaction necrosis does not create a barrier to penetration, and deep injury easily occurs. Alkali burns appear wet and may feel soapy to the touch.

Chemicals other than acids and alkali can cause corrosive damage and skin burns. Examples are phenol and related compounds, vesicants, alkylating agents, phosphorus, and alkaline metals. Fortunately, accidents with most of these chemicals are rare. Some of them will be discussed in detail later in this chapter.

DETERMINANTS OF SEVERITY

The severity of a chemical skin injury is determined by at least four separate factors.

1. Nature and reactivity of chemical

2. Concentration of the chemical

3. Integrity of skin

4. Duration of exposure

Nature and Reactivity of Chemical

Very reactive chemicals, particularly those that readily interact with the proteins or fatty substances of the skin, are most likely to cause serious injury and harm. In many cases, the dangers of the chemicals are obvious. For example, acids, alkali, and vesicants (blistering agents) are generally regarded as harmful to the skin. Conversely, the destructive effects of some commonly found chemicals may not be well known. For example, severe corrosive skin burns can result from prolonged contact with gasoline and other solvents. Likewise, Portland cement can produce severe skin burns.

Emergency responders should not assume that chemical skin contact is harmless. All victims who have suffered skin contamination should be thoroughly washed and decontaminated.

Concentration of Chemical

The concentration of a chemical can determine whether exposure will lead to mild irritation or serious skin burns. Concentrated acids and alkali produce intense skin burns when splashed on the skin. If they are diluted, however, they may cause only minor symptoms or none at all.

The same effects of concentration occur with irritant gases. At high air concentrations, gases such as chlorine, ammonia, and hydrogen chloride can cause severe irritation, dermatitis, and skin burns. At lower concentrations, exposure to those gases leads to only slight irritation and redness of the skin.

Concentration effects are important in determining how near unprotected persons can approach a hazardous materials incident. As gases and fumes spread downwind, they tend to dissipate, and air concentrations decrease. The farther away from the source of a gas leak, the lower will be the exposure risk. Clouds of gases can pose threats to life and health, however, even when they are no longer visible. In some cases, irritation of skin, eyes, and mucous membranes occurs more than a mile downwind.

Integrity of Skin

The severity of chemical-induced skin injury is increased when the skin and its barrier of corneum stratum are disrupted. For that reason, patients with abrasions or dermatitis are at increased risk following chemical skin exposures. Victims with lacerations and other open skin wounds are at even greater risk. Because those wounds remove all barriers to skin penetration, chemicals can freely enter and cause wound contamination; deep skin damage can result. Moreover, high levels of percutaneous absorption and systemic intoxication can occur when chemicals enter open wounds.

Duration of Exposure

Chemical exposure of the skin produces ongoing reactions that proceed until the chemical has been used up or removed from the skin. The amount of injury that results is directly related to the duration of skin exposure. This is a situation entirely different from thermal burns. Thermal burning stops once victims have been removed from the source of heat. By contrast, victims must be physically removed from the source of contamination *and* the chemical must be physically removed from the victim to stop chemical burning.

The importance of exposure duration has been often studied, generally by examining the effects of corrosive acids and alkali. Presented subsequently are the results of experiments demonstrating that prompt removal of corrosives, in most cases by washing with water, results in decreased tissue injury.

Application of acids or alkali to the skin causes large changes of the skin's pH, an indication of ongoing skin damage. Typical skin pH changes owing to strong solutions of hydrochloric acid and sodium hydroxide are shown in Figure 17–3. Also shown are the pH changes that result when skin exposure is promptly followed by washing in a water shower for up to 8 hours. Water is used to remove the corrosives from the skin and decrease the duration of exposure.

The alkali, sodium hydroxide, caused much greater and longer-lasting pH change than the acid. Moreover, the effects of sodium hydroxide remained despite continuous skin washing, whereas the acid effects quickly returned to normal. These experimental results, particularly the prolonged pH elevation after alkali exposure, suggest that alkali burns should be washed for hours to remove the alkali and limit exposure duration.

Studies in animals have repeatedly shown that if washing is initiated promptly, burns are less severe, and healing occurs more quickly. Studies have also shown that wiping away acids from the skin serves to limit the severity of skin burns. In some animal studies, the benefits of rapid removal of acids or alkali were only seen when washing began within a minute of skin exposure.

Humans cannot be subjected to experimental exposures. Much can be learned, however, by examining the clinical results for chemical burn patients admitted to hospital burn units. For example, Table 17–1 presents a comparison of the clinical outcomes of such patients grouped according to whether washing was promptly and adequately performed. Prompt washing was defined as washing begun within 10 minutes of exposure and adequate washing was defined as at least 15 minutes of continuous water irrigation.

These results demonstrate that although the properly washed burns were larger in total body surface area, they resulted in much fewer third-degree burns. Moreover, the patients who were promptly and adequately washed required much less time in the hospital than those in the inadequately washed group. These findings are a strong argument for the importance of quick, aggressive water irrigation of all corrosive skin exposures.

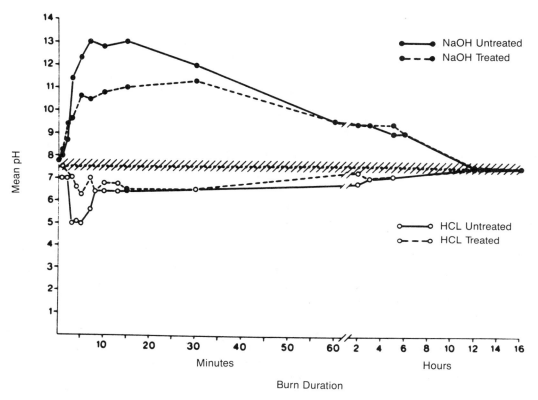

Figure 17–3 Effects of pH on dermis after application of sodium hydroxide, a powerful alkali, and hydrochloric acid. Effects of treatment (continuous washing of contaminated skin in a water shower) and no treatment are contrasted. Note that the pH change caused by the alkali is greater and longer lasting than that caused by acid. (From Gruber, R. P., D. R. Laub, and L. M. Vistnes, "The Effect of Hydrotherapy on the Clinical Course and pH of Experimental Cutaneous Chemical Burns," *Plast. Reconstr. Surg.*, 55 [1975], 2; reprinted with permission.)

Such clinical results emphasize that removal of chemicals from the skin is an essential first step in the emergency management of exposure victims. Skin washing must be initiated promptly and for a minimum of 15 minutes. In some cases, complete removal of chemicals may not be possible. That is more likely with alkali than acids and other corrosives. Unless other life-threatening conditions are present, victims should receive adequate washing before being transported by ambulance to a hospital or other health care center. When possible, irrigation should be continued during transport. A few chemicals exist, most notably water-reactive metals such as sodium and lithium, for which water washing should *not* be performed. Those chemicals are discussed in the last section of this chapter.

TABLE 17-1 CLINICAL VALUE OF PROPER SKIN WASHING
IN HOSPITALIZED CHEMICAL BURN PATIENTS*

	Prompt, adequate wash	Delayed or brief wash
No. of patients	37.0	46.0
Mean TBSA† burn	9.5%	7.1%
Third-degree burns	5 (13.5%)	28 (61%)
Mean hospital stay	6.2 days	22 days

*Adapted from Moran, K. D., T. O'Reilly, and A. M. Munster, "Chemical Burns: A Ten-Year Experience," *Am. Surg.*, 11 (1987), 652.
†TBSA = total body surface area.

COMPLICATIONS OF CHEMICAL SKIN BURNS

Victims of chemical skin burns are subject to many of the same complications that affect other victims of severe trauma. Like thermal burns, chemical burns can lead to dehydration because of fluid loss across the burned skin. These patients require aggressive fluid replacement by intravenous infusions. It is often difficult to judge the severity and size of a chemical burn until 48 hours or longer after the burn has occurred. Accordingly, a danger exists that chemical burn patients will receive too little fluid and will suffer dehydration and electrolyte abnormalities. Emergency responders should be careful not to underestimate the severity of a chemical burn.

Victims of chemical burns are also subject to many infectious complications including cellulitis, sepsis, pneumonia, and other potentially life-threatening infections. They can also suffer upper-gastrointestinal bleeding, kidney failure, and vascular emergencies such as myocardial infarctions. Table 17-2 presents the frequencies of some of these complications as reported for two large groups of chemical burn patients. Emergency responders must remember the high risk of life-threatening conditions in these victims.

CHEMICALS OF SPECIAL CONSIDERATION

A few chemicals require special management considerations or pose unique risks to rescuers. The following discussion provides a quick overview of some. Emergency responders who work in communities in which these chemicals are routinely used should consider developing specialized response protocols to assure that exposure victims receive appropriate care.

Hydrogen Fluoride

Hydrogen fluoride is an acidic and extremely corrosive substance. In water solutions it is known as hydrofluoric acid. Besides its effects as a potent acid, hydro-

TABLE 17–2 COMPLICATIONS OF CHEMICAL BURNS
IN HOSPITALIZED CHEMICAL BURN PATIENTS

Complication	Series A* (%) (n = 111)	Series B† (%) (n = 87)
Pneumonia	9	8
Cellulitis	5	10
Septicemia	5	9
Osteomyelitis	3	6
Upper GI‡ bleed	6	8
Acute renal failure	4	5

*Adapted from Curreri, P. W., M. J. Asch, and B. A. Pruitt,
"Treatment of Chemical Burns: Specialized Diagnostic, Therapeutic, and Prognostic Considerations," *J. Trauma*, 10 (1970),
634–41.

†Adapted from Mozinga, D. W., A. A. Smith, W. F. McManus,
et al., "Chemical Burns," *J. Trauma*, 28 (1988), 642–47.

‡GI = gastrointestinal.

gen fluoride binds to calcium and magnesium, making them unavailable to the cells of the body. Lack of calcium causes cell death. It can lead to seizures and cardiac rhythm abnormalities including fatal ventricular fibrillation. Death has been reported after burns involving only 2.5 percent of total body surface area.

The management of hydrogen fluoride burns includes administration of calcium salts. At many work sites that routinely use this chemical, calcium gluconate gel is used as the initial treatment after washing of hydrogen fluoride burns. Although not commercially available, this gel can be easily made by mixing 2.5 g of calcium gluconate USP in 100 ml of a water-soluble lubricant such as Surgilube or KY Jelly. The gel is applied to the burn site and rubbed into the skin while victims are transported to a medical facility. Use of this or similar management approaches should not be undertaken by EMS personnel without prior development of protocols and the approval of EMS medical control.

Phosphorus

Phosphorus is commonly found in military munitions and rat poison. Following explosions of phosphorus-containing munitions, victims may be sprayed by fine particles of molten phosphorus that penetrate the skin, and cause corrosive and thermal burns and systemic phosphorus absorption. Phosphorus ignites spontaneously in air at temperatures above 86°F to 90°F (30°C to 34°C). It will reignite itself after the fire has been extinguished if its temperature remains elevated. The vapors of burning phosphorus contain toxic gases that can cause further harm to exposed victims.

The first goal in caring for phosphorus burn victims is to extinguish burning and keep the temperature of the phosphorus below 86°F (30°C). The easiest way to do this is by submerging the burned part in cool water. During transport to a medical facility, the burned area should be covered with cool, moist dressings to prevent reignition of the phosphorus.

Water-Reactive Metals

The water-reactive metals, also called alkaline metals, include sodium, lithium, magnesium, and calcium. Skin exposed to these chemicals should not be washed with water. These chemicals react with water to yield heat and form strongly corrosive alkali. As a result, water exposure will lead to severer burns than if the skin had been kept dry.

Following skin contact, these metals can ignite. The fire should be smothered using sand or extinguished with class D fire extinguishers that are intended for this special use. Removal of imbedded pieces of metal requires surgical treatment. While transporting these victims to a medical facility, the burn area and imbedded metal can be covered with cooking oil. This procedure prevents the metal from making contact with the air and makes ignition less likely.

Phenol

Phenol (also called carbolic acid) and phenolic compounds are corrosive substances that are capable of causing fatal systemic poisoning. Skin contact can lead to severe chemical burns. Phenols are only slightly water soluble so that it is difficult to wash them from the skin with water. A more effective substance for removing phenols is polyethylene glycol, which allows rescuers to quickly wipe phenol off the skin. Polyethylene glycol is not generally available to EMS personnel, however, and specific protocols must be developed for its use when phenols are commonly used.

SUMMARY

Exposure to toxic chemicals can lead to skin injury and percutaneous absorption producing systemic poisoning. The severity of injury is often determined by the duration of toxic exposure. Prompt and thorough removal of toxic substances from the skin is an essential first step in the care of exposure victims. In most cases, this is accomplished by copious water washing.

Chemical skin burns can lead to severe complications, like those associated with severe trauma. Rescuers must not underestimate the severity or extent of burns. Intravenous fluids are generally required to prevent burn victims from developing dehydration and electrolyte disorders.

Some chemicals pose unique problems or require special management to minimize injury to victims. In communities in which such chemicals are routinely used, it is useful to develop specific EMS protocols that allow medically approved emergency care of victims.

REFERENCES

Anon., *First Aid Treatment for Hydrofluoric Acid Burns.* Morristown, N.J.: Allied-Signal, 1987.

BRONSTEIN, A. C., and P. L. CURRANCE, *Emergency Care for Hazardous Materials Exposure.* St. Louis: The C. V. Mosby Company, 1988.

BROWN, V. K. H., V. L. BOX, and B. J. SIMPSON, "Decontamination Procedures for Skin Exposed to Phenolic Substances," *Arch. Environ. Health,* 30 (1975), 1–6.

BUCKLEY, D. D., "Skin Burns due to Wet Cement," *Contact Dermatitis,* 8 (1982), 407–9.

CURRERI, P. W., M. J. ASCH, and B. A. PRUITT, "Treatment of Chemical Burns: Specialized Diagnostic, Therapeutic, and Prognostic Considerations," *J. Trauma,* 10 (1970), 634–41.

EMMETT, E. A., "Toxic Responses of the Skin," in *Casarett and Doull's Toxicology: The Basic Science of Poisons,* pp. 412–31, eds. C. D. Klaassen, M. O. Amdur, and J. Doull. New York: Macmillan Publishing Co., Inc., 1986.

FITZPATRICK, K. T., and J. A. MOYLAN, "Emergency Care of Chemical Burns," *Postgrad. Med. J.,* 78 (1985), 189–94.

GRUBER, R. P., D. R. LAUB, and L. M. VISTNES, "Effect of Hydrotherapy on the Clinical Course and pH of Experimental Cutaneous Chemical Burns," *Plast. Reconstr. Surg.,* 55 (1975), 200–4.

JELENKO, C., "Chemicals that 'Burn'," *J. Trauma,* 14 (1974), 65–72.

KONJOYAN, T. R., "White Phosphorus Burns: Case Report and Literature Review," *Milit. Med.,* 148 (1983), 881–84.

LEONARD, G., J. J. SCHEULEN, and A. M. MUNSTER, "Chemical Burns: Effect of Prompt First Aid," *J. Trauma,* 22 (1982), 420–23.

MORAN, K. D., T. O'REILLY, and A. M. MUNSTER, "Chemical Burns: A Ten-Year Experience," *Am. Surg.,* 11 (1987), 652–53.

MOZINGO, D. W., A. A. SMITH, W. F. MCMANUS, et al., "Chemical Burns," *J. Trauma,* 28 (1988), 642–47.

RODHEAVER, G. T., J. M. HIEBERT, and R. F. EDLICH, "Initial Treatment of Chemical Skin and Eye Burns," *Compr. Ther.,* 8 (1982), 37–43.

STEWART, C. E., "Chemical Skin Burns," *Am. Fam. Physician,* 31 (1985), 149–57.

VAN RENSBURG, L. C. J., "Experimental Chemical Burns," *South African Med. J.,* 36 (1962), 754–59.

WALSH, W. A., F. J. SCARPA, R. S. BROWN, et al., "Gasoline Immersion Burn," *N. Engl. J. Med.,* 291 (1974), 830.

WHITE, J. W., "Hydrofluoric Acid Burns," *Cutis* 34 (1984), 241–44.

ACUTE SYSTEMIC INTOXICATIONS

CHAPTER 18

GOAL: On completion of this chapter the student will have an understanding of the ways in which hazardous materials can be absorbed systemically and will understand the mechanisms by which they can cause life-threatening emergencies.

OBJECTIVES:

Specifically, the student will be able to

- Describe the routes of exposure that lead to systemic absorption and poisoning by hazardous materials
- Explain why some chemicals cause systemic effects rapidly after absorption, whereas others have a much slower onset of action
- List four ways that chemicals can cause asphyxia in an exposure victim and describe the types of chemicals that have asphyxiant effects
- Describe the effects that absorbed chemicals can have on the CNS, and name some common medical conditions that cause similar CNS effects
- Describe the characteristic clinical effects of neurotoxic insecticides
- Explain how exposure to toxic chemicals can cause life-threatening electrolyte disorders

OVERVIEW

This chapter addresses toxic effects that occur after harmful chemicals have been absorbed and circulated through the bloodstream. First, the routes of exposure leading to systemic intoxication are considered. Then, factors determining rate of onset are discussed. Finally, types of systemic intoxication likely to be encountered by rescuers at hazardous materials incidents are described.

The previous three chapters were concerned with toxic effects involving organs that make direct contact with harmful chemicals in our environment. Particular attention was given to toxic injuries of the lung, skin, and eye. Such injuries are examples of localized toxic effects. The affected organs can be described as targets of those harmful chemicals.

By contrast, the toxic effects of concern here involve organs that are not directly exposed to harmful environmental chemicals. Those harmful chemicals must first enter the body and then be distributed to the organs that are harmed. Toxic effects result from systemic, rather than localized, exposure. In some cases, systemic exposure leads to toxicity of all the body's cells. In others, harm is caused only to specific organs. We can speak of organs that are especially vulnerable as the targets of systemic intoxication.

ROUTES OF EXPOSURE

Chemicals can be absorbed following inhalation or contact with skin and eye. Inhalation is the commonest exposure route leading to systemic toxicity. Relatively large amounts of many types of chemicals can be rapidly absorbed from inhaled air as it passes through the nose, pharynx, and airways into the alveoli. Both water-soluble and fat-soluble compounds can be taken up into the systemic circulation.

In general, chemicals that cause immediate, localized injury to the airways and lungs are poorly absorbed. The reason for this may be due to reactions between those chemicals and lung tissue. As a result, the chemicals bind to the tissues and become unavailable to be absorbed. Alternatively, it is possible that chemical-induced lung damage alters the lung so that absorption cannot occur. By contrast, chemicals that cause few localized effects are often well absorbed from the lungs.

Absorption of chemicals from the skin, or *percutaneous absorption,* is another important exposure route leading to systemic intoxication. As discussed in chapter 9, the corneum stratum is a layer of dead cells that covers the skin and acts as a barrier that prevents chemical contact and absorption. Fat-soluble substances penetrate that barrier more easily than water-soluble compounds and are more readily absorbed. Disruptions of the corneum stratum, such as abrasions and open skin wounds, increase percutaneous absorption of most chemicals. Other factors that influence the quantity of percutaneous chemical absorption include the concentration of the applied chemical, duration of exposure, surface area exposed, amount of skin moisture, and skin temperature. Moist, warm skin absorbs chemicals more effectively than cool, dry skin.

Chemicals can also be absorbed from the eye, although the quantities absorbed are usually small. In animal studies, however, several drops of hydrogen cyanide applied to the cornea resulted in absorption, systemic intoxication, and death. It is not known whether similar toxic effects could result in humans.

ONSET OF ACTION

The effects of systemic intoxication may occur immediately after exposure or may be delayed for days or longer. The rate of *onset of action* depends in part on whether the chemical is toxic in the form that is absorbed. Many chemicals are themselves nearly harmless but are transformed in the body to agents that cause severe harm. Chemicals that are harmful without such transformation usually cause a rapid onset of effects. Those that require transformation to be toxic, conversely, are associated with more delayed effects.

This is illustrated by the contrast between hydrogen cyanide and acrylonitrile, an important industrial chemical that is transformed to yield hydrogen cyanide. Following absorption, hydrogen cyanide is immediately toxic. It requires no transformation to exert its effects on the body's cells. Symptoms can develop within seconds and death within minutes after large-dose inhalations. Acrylonitrile causes the same toxic effects as cyanide and is just as lethal. The effects of acrylonitrile, however, may not develop for hours or longer after exposure. The difference in onset of actions is due to the need to transform acrylonitrile before toxicity can occur.

Some chemicals cause both immediate and delayed effects. The immediate effects are usually due to the chemical in the form that has been absorbed. The delayed effects result from transformation products. Methanol is an example of a chemical with both immediate and delayed systemic effects. Following exposure, a rapid onset of toxic effects such as ethanol-like drunkenness occurs. Those effects are directly due to untransformed methanol. By contrast, visual changes and blindness, the most characteristic toxic effects of methanol poisoning, do not develop for 12 to 30 hours after exposure. They are not caused by methanol itself, but by formic acid that is a product of methanol metabolism. Visual toxicity does not develop until a large amount of formic acid has accumulated. By the time blindness develops, usually little if any methanol is left in the victim's body.

In unusual cases, hazardous chemicals cause delayed effects. For example, neurological and psychiatric disturbances have been reported to develop months or years after exposure to methyl chloride, a refrigerant gas. It is also believed that tumors and cancers can result years after acute exposures to chemicals such as benzene, although some disagreement exists about whether this actually can happen after a single, acute exposure.

Delayed effects of these sorts are rarely important to EMS clinical care because such effects develop long after the emergency has been managed. Such effects, however, might develop and cause illness to emergency responders who were exposed while performing a rescue. For this reason, responders involved in hazardous materials incidents should undergo regular, periodic medical examinations and routine laboratory testing (see Appendix 4). It is also advised that responders keep a diary in which they record all exposures or contaminations that they have suffered. This diary should include the names of chemicals causing exposure, the date of the exposure, and any symptoms that developed. This information should then be made available to the responder's personal physician.

ASPHYXIANTS

Exposure to hazardous chemicals can cause *asphyxia,* a condition in which the cells are deprived of oxygen. Asphyxia can rapidly lead to death or severe damage of organs that are particularly sensitive to oxygen deficiency. Such organs are the CNS, liver, and kidneys. Several different mechanisms exist by which toxic chemicals can produce cellular oxygen deficiency and asphyxia.

1. Inhibition of cellular respiration
2. Production of abnormal hemoglobin
3. Acute hemolysis
4. Interference with ventilation

Inhibition of Cellular Respiration

Cellular respiration, the process by which cells make use of oxygen, consists of a sequence of intracellular reactions that are each controlled by specific enzymes. The most important and sensitive of those enzymes is *cytochrome oxidase.* Interference with that enzyme, either by reducing its quantity or blocking its function, inhibits the ability of the cells to use oxygen. When that occurs, the cells are deprived of oxygen, a condition known as *intracellular hypoxia.*

Several chemicals can interact with and block cytochrome oxidase and thereby cause intracellular hypoxia. The best known are hydrogen cyanide and hydrogen sulfide, both of which bind to cytochrome oxidase molecules. The effects of these chemicals can be rapid, sometimes causing unconsciousness in seconds and death within minutes. In addition, cyanide is released slowly by the metabolism of cyanide-containing compounds, notably nitriles and cyanohydrins, leading to toxicity with delayed onset.

The clinical signs and physical findings observed in these victims are nonspecific, and diagnosis may be difficult. Victims at first seem anxious and often hyperventilate. Later, severe dyspnea without cyanosis is present. A history of exposure is usually necessary to allow a correct diagnosis to be made promptly, and rescuers must aggressively seek such a history. These patients should receive supplemental oxygen; however, medical treatment with antidotes is usually necessary to prevent fatal outcomes.

Production of Abnormal Hemoglobin

Some chemicals interact with the hemoglobin in red blood cells. Hemoglobin is a protein that carries oxygen from the lungs to the body's cells. When chemical interactions decrease the ability of hemoglobin to carry oxygen, cells suffer acute oxygen deficiency. Carbon monoxide is the best known chemical that decreases the oxygen-carrying ability of blood by converting normal hemoglobin to *carboxyhemoglobin*. Carboxyhemoglobin formation usually results from carbon monoxide inhalation, but some victims have developed this condition following exposure to methylene chloride, a solvent used in paint removers and other industrial products. Victims complain of headache, weakness, nausea, and dizziness. Unconsciousness, seizures, myocardial infarction, cerebral infarction, and death can occur. The blood is usually very red and healthy in appearance, and no evidence of cyanosis is present. Management of these victims requires aggressive administration of oxygen.

Another form of abnormal hemoglobin results from chemicals that can oxidize hemoglobin to *methemoglobin*, a form of hemoglobin that cannot carry oxygen. Methemoglobin causes the blood to appear chocolate brown in color and victims often suffer deep cyanosis. Methemoglobin can be produced by many chemicals, especially nitrogen-containing compounds such as nitrites and amines. These victims require supplemental oxygen. For severe exposure, medical treatment with antidotes such as methylene blue is often necessary.

Acute Hemolysis

Acute exposure to some chemicals causes sudden, acute destruction of red blood cells, or *hemolysis*. Hemolysis can result in anemia so severe that the tissues do not receive adequate amounts of oxygen. One chemical known to cause acute, severe hemolysis is arsine. That chemical is used in the manufacture of computer chips. It is also released spontaneously during some metallurgical processes. Hemolysis usually develops several hours following exposure. Victims require supplemental oxygen and prompt medical evaluation.

Interference with Ventilation

Heavier-than-air gases can displace oxygen, resulting in asphyxiation because air cannot enter the lungs. This can occur when a heavy gas leaks into and fills a room, engulfing and strangling people in that room. It can also occur when an unconscious victim's lungs are filled by such a gas so that oxygen cannot enter the lungs. These exposures are similar to drowning; they are caused by gases and not by liquids. Management requires ventilation with oxygen after the victims have been removed from the contaminated place.

CENTRAL NERVOUS SYSTEM DEPRESSANTS

Depression of the CNS leading to anesthetic and narcotic effects can be caused by many hazardous chemicals. Examples include alcohols (such as methanol and butanol), aromatic hydrocarbons (such as benzene and toluene), ketones (such as methyl ethyl ketone), and halogenated hydrocarbons (such as carbon tetrachloride and methyl chloride). Most are fat-soluble compounds that accumulate and reach high concentrations in the fatty tissues of the brain. The mechanisms by which these compounds cause their effects are not certain, but one possibility involves effects on the membranes of nerve cells.

The clinical effects caused by exposure are determined by a chemical's activity and the exposure dose. Mild effects, caused by exposure to low doses and weak agents include drunkenness, dulled thinking, and drowsiness. Moderate effects include loss of coordination, stumbling gait, and slurred speech. Severe effects are due to high-dose exposures and potent agents. Such exposures lead to loss of consciousness, coma, respiratory arrest, seizures, and death. These victims can be confused with patients suffering common medical conditions such as ethanol or drug intoxication, uncontrolled diabetes, hypoglycemia, cerebrovascular accidents, epilepsy, dehydration, meningitis, and hysteria.

The first priority of emergency management is to assure adequate ventilation and oxygenation. Even deeply comatose patients can survive if ventilation is maintained. As described subsequently, many of these agents can sensitize the heart and predispose to ventricular fibrillation. Therefore, these victims should be kept at rest and closely monitored. Victims with evidence of CNS depression require medical evaluation to rule out the presence of underlying disease.

CARDIAC SENSITIZERS

Several chemicals sensitize the heart to epinephrine and related *catecholamines*. Catecholamines are substances produced by the body such as epinephrine (adrenaline) and dopamine, which increase the heart rate and blood pressure. They are released normally as part of the body's response to stress and fear, a process sometimes called the ''flight or fight'' response. Sensitization of the heart to catecholamines causes increased cardiac response to stress. In particular, a danger exists that catecholamine stimulation will cause ventricular fibrillation, cardiac arrest, and death in exposure victims.

Chemicals known to sensitize the heart in this way include many commonly used solvents and hydrocarbons such as benzene, toluene, and trichloroethylene. Catecholamine release in victims may be stimulated by anxiety and fear. When possible, victims who have been exposed to solvents and hydrocarbons should be observed using cardiac monitors. They should be kept at rest until medically evaluated. If medical indications to administer catecholamines to these patients exist (for example, the use of epinephrine during cardiac resuscitation or dopamine for hypotension and shock), then smaller-than-standard doses should be given.

NEUROTOXIC INSECTICIDES

Pesticides are a group of highly toxic chemicals that are deliberately used because of their ability to kill. Although intended to injure rodents, insects, and other pests that damage crops and foodstuffs or spread disease, these agents are also capable of causing severe harm to humans. The pesticides most commonly associated with human exposure and disease are insecticides of the type known as *organophosphates.* Similar but slightly less toxic are the insecticides known as *carbamates.*

Organophosphate and carbamate insecticides directly affect the nervous system. This group of insecticides include the chemical warfare agents known as nerve gases. Many different organophosphates and carbamates have been commercially developed. Some examples are parathion, diazinon, and aldicarb. They act by blocking *cholinesterase,* an enzyme that is critical to maintaining the normal functions of the *parasympathetic nervous system.* Exposure to organophosphates and carbamates leads to excessive parasympathetic activity. Among the effects of parasympathetic stimulation are slowing of the heart rate, bronchospasm and asthma, increased gastrointestinal activity, contraction of the bladder, salivation, and tear formation.

A characteristic set of clinical effects is caused by toxic exposure to these insecticides, which usually include the following:

- Bradycardia leading to heart block
- Chest tightness and wheezing
- Increased salivation, sweating, and lacrimation
- Increased urination
- Abdominal cramps with nausea and vomiting
- Constricted pupils
- Weakness, twitching, muscle tremors, and cramps

Severe exposure leads to seizures, coma, circulatory collapse, respiratory arrest, and death. The onset of symptoms can occur within minutes or may be delayed for several hours. Symptoms can last for up to five days. In fatal cases, death usually occurs during the first 24 hours.

These insecticides can be rapidly fatal. Fortunately, their toxic effects are so characteristic that early diagnosis is usually possible. The first priority of management is to assure adequate ventilation. Careful decontamination with soap and water and removal of all contaminated clothing and leather goods is essential. Percutaneous absorption is an important route of exposure for these chemicals. Medical treatment with large doses of atropine, which blocks the insecticides' effects, is usually required. Because atropine is commonly available as a cardiac resuscitation medication in paramedic EMS services, it is often possible to begin antidotal treatment while victims are being transported to definitive medical care facilities. Prompt treatment with atropine is often indicated but must not be given without medical approval.

ELECTROLYTE DISORDERS

Potentially life-threatening electrolyte disorders can result from exposure to toxic chemicals. Examples are toxins such as hydrogen fluoride, oxalic acid, and phosphorus, which act as *sequestration agents* that bind calcium. Calcium is essential for many cellular functions including normal control of the heart and nervous system. Depletion of calcium leads to low blood calcium concentrations, or *hypocalcemia.*

Hypocalcemia causes hyperactivity of the central and peripheral nervous systems, leading to twitching, muscle spasms, and seizures. Disturbances of the heart rhythm and cardiac arrest can also result. Deaths resulting from hypocalcemia have been reported in victims suffering relatively small burns caused by phosphorus or hydrofluoric acid. Measurement of electrolytes in the blood should be carried out in every patient who has suffered toxic exposures to these agents.

Cardiac rhythm disturbances have also been described in patients who have absorbed large amounts of lithium following skin exposure. Exposure to a related metal, calcium, can lead to abnormal cardiac rhythms because of increased blood levels of calcium (or *hypercalcemia*). Because patients with active metal burns generally require surgical treatment, these patients should all be transported to definitive medical care facilities where appropriate blood testing can be performed.

Severe acidosis can result from acute toxic exposures. This has occurred after inhalation of chlorine and skin exposure to hydrochloric acid. Profound acidosis is also an important aspect of the intoxication caused by methanol. Severe acidosis can lead to hyperventilation, similar to Kussmaul respirations seen in diabetic ketoacidosis, shock, and cardiac rhythm disturbances. Ventricular fibrillation and cardiac arrest may result.

SUMMARY

Systemic intoxications can follow toxic exposures caused by inhalation, or contact with the skin and eye. Clinical effects may develop immediately or after a delay. Because some systemic effects do not develop for months or years following exposure, emergency responders should maintain a diary in which they keep a record of their exposure histories. Those responders should undergo regular, periodic medical examinations. Exposure diaries should be made available to their physicians.

Among the many forms of systemic intoxication that can be caused by hazardous materials, only a few are likely to be of clinical importance to rescuers. Among those are asphyxiant reactions, CNS depression, cardiac sensitization leading to cardiac dysrhythmias, neurotoxicity caused by insecticides, and electrolyte disorders leading to cardiac and neurological dysfunction.

Emergency responders should be aware of the possibility of systemic intoxication. For most of these victims, maintaining ventilation, close observation, and rapid transport to a medical facility are the primary goals of EMS response.

REFERENCES

AMMANN, H. M., "New Look at Physiologic Respiratory Response to H₂S Poisoning," *J. Haz. Mat.*, 13 (1986), 369–74.

BAKINSON, M. A., and R. D. JONES, "Gassings due to Methylene Chloride, Xylene, Toluene, and Styrene Reported to Her Majesty's Factory Inspectorate 1961–80," *Br. J. Ind. Med.*, 42 (1985), 184–90.

BASS, M., "Sudden Sniffing Death," *JAMA*, 212 (1970), 2075–79.

BEAUCHAMP, R. O., J. A. POPP, and C. J. BOREIKO, et al., "Critical Review of the Literature on Hydrogen Sulfide Toxicity," *CRC Crit. Rev. Toxicol.*, 13 (1984), 25–97.

BOWEN, T. E., T. J. WHELAN, and T. G. NELSON, "Sudden Death after Phosphorus Burns: Experimental Observations of Hypocalcemia, Hyperphosphatemia and Electrocardiographic Abnormalities following Production of a Standard White Phosphorus Burn," *Ann. Surg.*, 174 (1971), 779–84.

BRONSTEIN, A. C., and P. L CURRANCE, *Emergency Care for Hazardous Materials Exposure.* St.Louis: The C. V. Mosby Company, 1988.

CUMMINGS, C . C., and M. E. McIVOR, "Fluoride-Induced Hyperkalemia," *Am. J. Emerg. Med.*, 6 (1988), 1–3.

CUSHMAN, P., and B. H. ALEXANDER, "Renal Phosphate and Calcium Excretory Defects in a Case of Acute Phosphorus Poisoning," *Nephron*, 3 (1966), 123–28.

DIBBELL, DAVID G., RONALD E. IVERSON, and WALLACE JONES, et al., "Hydrofluoric Acid Burns of the Hand," *J. Bone Joint Surg.*, 52A (1970), 931–36.

EMMETT, E. A., "Toxic Responses of the Skin," in *Casarett and Doull's Toxicology: The Basic Science of Poisons*, pp. 412–31, eds. C. D. Klaassen, M. O. Amdur, and J. Doull. New York: Macmillan Publishing Co., Inc., 1986.

ENGER, E., "Acidosis, Gaps and Poisonings" [editorial], *Acta Med. Scand.*, 212 (1982), 1–3.

GUDMUNDSSON, G., "Methyl Chloride Poisoning 13 Years Later," *Arch. Environ. Health*, 32 (1977), 236–37.

HALL, A. H., and B. H. RUMACK, "Clinical Toxicology of Cyanide," *Ann. Emerg. Med.*, 15 (1986), 1067–73.

KAPLAN, K., "Methyl Alcohol Poisoning," *Am. J. Med. Sci.*, 76 (1962), 170–74.

KEGEL, A. H., W. D. MCNALLY, and A. S. POPE, "Methyl Chloride Poisoning from Domestic Refrigerators," *JAMA*, 93 (1929), 353–58.

MENCHEL, S. M., and W. A. DUNN, "Hydrofluoric Acid Poisoning," *Am. J. Forensic Med. Pathol.*, 5 (1984), 245–48.

MENZEL, D. B., and M. O. AMDUR, "Toxic Responses of the Respiratory System," in *Casarett and Doull's Toxicology: The Basic Science of Poisons*, pp. 330–58, eds. C. D. Klaassen, M. O. Amdur, and J. Doull. New York: Macmillan Publishing Co., Inc., 1986.

MORGAN, D. P., *Recognition and Management of Pesticide Poisonings*. Washington, D.C.: U.S. Environmental Protection Agency, 1982.

MURPHY, S. D., "Toxic Effects of Pesticides," in *Casarett and Doull's Toxicology: The Basic Science of Poisons*, pp. 519–81, eds. C. D. Klaassen, M. O. Amdur, and J. Doull. New York: Macmillan Publishing Co., Inc., 1986.

NORTON, S., "Toxic Responses of the Central Nervous System," in *Casarett and Doull's Toxicology: The Basic Science of Poisons*, pp. 359–86, eds. C. D. Klaassen, M. O. Amdur, and J. Doull. New York: Macmillan Publishing Co., Inc., 1986.

O'DONOGHUE, J. L., "Aliphatic Halogenated Hydrocarbons, Alcohols, and Acids and Thioacids," in *Neurotoxicity of Industrial and Commercial Chemicals* (vol. 2), pp. 99–126, ed. J. L. O'Donoghue. Boca Raton, Fla.: CRC Press, 1985.

O'DONOGHUE, J. L., "Alkanes, Alcohols, Ketones, and Ethylene Oxide," in *Neurotoxicity of Industrial and Commercial Chemicals* (vol. 2), pp. 61–97, ed. J. L. O'Donoghue. Boca Raton, Fla.: CRC Press, 1985.

O'DONOGHUE, J. L., "Aromatic Hydrocarbons," in *Neurotoxicity of Industrial and Commercial Chemicals* (vol. 2), pp. 127–37, ed. J. L. O'Donoghue. Boca Raton, Fla.: CRC Press, 1985.

POTTS, A. M., "Toxic Responses of the Eye," in *Casarett and Doull's Toxicology: The Basic Science of Poisons*, pp. 478–515, eds. C. D. Klaassen, M. O. Amdur, and J. Doull. New York: Macmillan Publishing Co., Inc., 1986.

REINHARDT, C. F., A. AZAR, and M. E. MAXFIELD, et al., "Cardiac Arrhythmias and Aerosol 'Sniffing'," *Arch. Environ. Health*, 22 (1971), 265–79.

REINHARDT, C. F., L. S. MULLIN, and M. E. MAXFIELD, "Epinephrine-Induced Cardiac Arrhythmia Potential of Some Common Industrial Solvents," *J. Occup. Med.*, 15 (1973), 953–55.

SEJERSTED, O. M., D. JACOBSEN, and S. OVREBO, et al., "Formate Concentrations in Plasma from Patients Poisoned with Methanol," *Acta Med. Scand.*, 213 (1983), 105–10.

SMITH, R. P., "Toxic Responses of the Blood," in *Casarett and Doull's Toxicology: The Basic Science of Poisons,* pp. 223–44, eds. C. D. Klaassen, M. O. Amdur, and J. Doull. New York: Macmillan Publishing Co., Inc., 1986.

TAHER, S. M., R. J. ANDERSON, and R. MCCARTNEY, et al., "Renal Tubular Acidosis Associated with Toluene 'Sniffing'," *N. Engl. J. Med.,* 290 (1974), 765–68.

TANII, H., and K. HASHIMOTO, "Structure-Acute Toxicity Relationship of Dinitriles in Mice," *Arch. Toxicol.,* 57 (1985), 88–93.

TEPHLY, T. R., K. E. MCMARTIN, "Methanol Metabolism and Toxicity," *Food Sci. Tech.,* 12 (1984), 111–40.

TEPPERMAN, PAUL B., "Fatality due to Acute Systemic Fluoride Poisoning Following a Hydrofluoric Acid Skin Burn," *J. Occup. Med.,* 22 (1980), 691–92.

VANCE, MICHAEL V., STEVEN C. CURRY, and DONALD B. KUNKEL, et al., "Digital Hydrofluoric Acid Burns: Treatment with Intraarterial Calcium Infusion," *Ann. Emerg. Med.,* 15 (1986), 890–96.

WAY, J. L., "Cyanide Intoxication and Its Mechanism of Antagonism," *Ann. Rev. Pharmacol. Toxicol.,* 24 (1984), 451–81.

WILLHITE, C. C., and R. P. SMITH, "The Role of Cyanide Liberation in the Acute Toxicity of Aliphatic Nitriles," *Toxicol. Appl. Pharmacol.,* 59 (1981), 589–602.

EMERGENCY RESPONDERS AND STRESS

Larry M. Starr, Ph.D.   **CHAPTER 19**

__GOAL:__   On completion of this chapter the student will understand the phenomenon of psychological stress and techniques for coping with stress reactions.

__OBJECTIVES:__

Specifically, the student will be able to

- Describe the two stages of stress
- Describe the three general categories of stressors
- Describe the three levels of stress preparation and intervention

OVERVIEW

Rescue efforts at hazardous materials incidents involve risks to more than just the physical well-being of rescuers; threats to the short- and long-term *psychological* health of EMS and other response personnel also occur. These emergencies can act as "critical incidents," specific events or situations capable of evoking unusually strong emotional reactions. It is as ill advised to enter a hazardous materials scene without education about potential psychological responses to the hazardous setting as it would be without prior education and training about the potential physical health risks.

Three psychological concerns of particular importance are as follows:

1. The signs and symptoms of emotional effects are not always immediately apparent. They can develop in subtle forms hours, days, or even months after the original event has occurred.

243

2. Physical injuries and illnesses generally develop in a dose-related fashion. For that reason, they are most likely to develop in victims who have suffered the greatest exposure. Psychological distress, conversely, evolves in a less systematic way. The likely victims of psychological distress are difficult to predict. For example, a seasoned rescuer with mild exposure may experience severer psychological reactions than does a novice responder with heavy contamination.

3. The results of psychological injury can be severe. In some cases, previously good rescuers suddenly quit. Others remain on the job, unwilling or unable to acknowledge openly that they are experiencing emotional distress, giving an ''unaccountably'' poor performance. A few become clinically depressed or even commit suicide.

This chapter will first address the psychological aspects of hazardous materials planning and responses. Concepts that explain the ways in which we react to stress and the sorts of concerns that produce stress are described. Also considered are some of the signs, symptoms, and behaviors of stress reactions. Then a technique is discussed that is currently used to reduce stress and cope with stress reactions that can interfere with EMS effectiveness.

STRESS

Stress is a complex process that can be divided into at least two stages. First, stress is said to occur when we are aroused by a challenge or threat related to psychological or environmental events. Receiving an emergency call from a plant where a colleague was severely injured by a chemical exposure during a previous run can produce pressure or stress in a rescuer. Responding for the first time to a site where it is known that severely toxic substances are used or stored can also produce stress. This initial stage of stress involves the anticipation of a threat or risk and leads to efforts to adapt or cope. Often, we are unaware of the initial part of this process: The pager or tone alarm goes off, and automatic responses occur. This description involves successful coping; the challenge is eliminated or minimized. Aside from an immediate, initial increase in arousal that drops away quickly, no permanent distress or anxiety occurs.

The second stage of stress involves the actual responses made to manage the arousal created by the threats associated with the first stage. This occurs when coping is not automatically successful and a concerted effort is needed to act in a controlled manner. When we believe that the probability of danger in a situation is high and that routine responses may not be adequate to cope with those dangers, then psychological and physical changes are evoked. Examples are known as the ''flight or fight'' reactions, and are associated with increased adrenal, cardiovascular, and respiratory function. A hazardous materials rescue scene can create such stress responses. As described in earlier chapters, in some situations rescuers must spend a great deal of thought and energy to assure their own safety before providing care to victims. EMS personnel, accustomed and trained to provide immediate care, may not be able to respond in a customarily rapid fashion. This can require that they work extra hard to control their stress in situations that can be both frightening and enormously frustrating. If efforts to cope remain unsuccessful, arousal is not reduced and decision making and personal health can suffer.

One difficulty in understanding and predicting the effects of stress is that they cannot be related simply to the situation alone. The same event can affect different people in different ways depending on personality and previous experience and conditioning. One important psychological issue that influences the degree of stress is whether the rescuer feels the situation is threatening. Regardless of how justified the judgment or whether others agree with us, when we *anticipate* that a threat will exist, stress follows. When serious personal risk, anxiety, or conflict are felt, people behave in various ways ranging from rationality to panic. Because we do not all feel the same way about all emergency calls, profound differences in the levels of stress are often experienced by different people at the same emergency scene.

TYPES OF STRESSORS

The term *stressor* is often used when we refer to events that actually produce stress in us. Three general categories of stressors can affect EMS hazardous materials incident responders.

Background stressors are the everyday, routine kinds of hassles and annoyances that are a ''part of the job.'' These include job dissatisfaction, equipment inadequacy or failure, political problems, unnecessary dispatches in the middle of the night, death and dying, and at-the-scene insensitivities. Although these are of relatively low intensity and by themselves do not usually pose important health risks to the persons who experience them, their cumulative effects can be upsetting. Their impact persists indefinitely, creating stress responses that are chronic.

Such forces are often in the background of one's job and may or may not be shared by all squad members. Even when they are shared, adequate coping or adaptation may not occur because the solution is beyond the direct control of the individual members of the group.

Personal stressors are more individualized and have more severe consequences. A few common examples include responses to family illness or disruption, problems of money and other forms of security, and issues about love and personal goals. These powerful forces can seriously hinder job performance. Because they can preoccupy and distract a rescuer, they can lead to errors in decision making and a lack of attention to responsibilities at the scene.

Coping efforts are sometimes as demanding and disrupting as the stresses themselves. Some examples of extreme sorts of behavior that may result from coping efforts include depending on alcohol and drugs, or throwing oneself into work as an escape from the disruptive effects of personal stressors. Typically, we deal with personal stressors by talking with friends and others. We make comparisons between ourselves and our co-workers and friends in an effort to gain positive feedback, and thereby decrease the intensity of the stresses we feel. Unfortunately, these techniques often do not produce solutions to the problems that provoked the stress nor do they eliminate the stress-related symptoms.

Cataclysmic events are generally universal in their effects. They require much effort to cope and may lead to immediate or long-term aftereffects. Mass casualty incidents on the streets can produce considerable stress, but chemical disasters go much beyond that in their stress-producing capabilities. Many adjustments in standard operating procedures must occur and, often, coordination with various unfamiliar people at the scene is required. These changes, added to the severe personal hazards of the rescue efforts, create enormous anxiety in everyone involved. Although it is sometimes assumed that EMS responders enjoy these exciting and dangerous events, the psychological hazards associated with chemical accidents can easily overwhelm personal limits and cause serious life disruptions that do not quickly fade.

Being emotionally overwhelmed does not necessarily require a catastrophic event, although such occurrences are likely to create extremely strong stress responses. Even a small event can create a severe stress response in people with high pre-existing levels of personal and background stressors. Such people may not have the ''strength'' to cope with a major disaster. Similarly, when a cataclysmic event is over and has taxed the rescuer to his or her limit, the additional effects of personal or background stressors, which would normally have been easily managed, can become intolerable.

STRESS DEBRIEFING PROCESS

Successful management of the stresses that develop in participants at a hazardous materials rescue effort requires the following three levels of preparation and intervention:

1. Preincident planning and education

2. At-the-scene intervention

3. Postincident management

One useful technique for presenting the subject of EMS responder stress as a topic appropriate for formal training and education is critical incident stress debriefing (CISD). CISD is an educational and psychological procedure of support that uses group discussions with specially trained EMS responders and health care professionals who serve as discussion group leaders. The main objective is to reduce the distress experienced as a result of the hazardous material (or any other critical) incident and to increase the likelihood of a return to routine functioning as soon as possible. To be most effective, management of psychological stress responses should be started before a critical incident has occurred.

CISD is not psychotherapy, and it does not deal directly with cases of "post-traumatic stress syndrome." For individuals who develop very severe levels of stress, there may be a need for psychotherapy or other interventions which go beyond the scope of CISD.

Preincident Planning and Education

All emergency responders should be knowledgeable about the causes and effects of stress. Education and training sessions on stress and its management should be made available to EMS personnel as part of the continuing education programs that most EMS systems provide. In particular, responders need to learn about and recognize their own reactions to stress. In most cases, the earliest stress-related symptoms are mostly internal (for example, loss of concentration, memory lapses, nausea, or anxiety) and are not generally apparent to command officers or co-workers until work performance has been disrupted. The likelihood that levels of stress will continue to rise until individual performances are compromised is increased when signs and symptoms of stress reactions are not recognized and promptly addressed.

With continued activity at the scene, stressed responders attempt to cope to maintain levels of function. If unsuccessful, however, stress reactions can seriously interfere with personal and victim safety. Simple procedures for assessment or management of victims may be forgotten, reflexes may be slow, and distraction and confusion may increase. Excessive stress is usually the reason that co-workers begin to act in unexpected ways, and demonstrate "strange" or inappropriate behavior at the scene of emergencies that require concentration and strict adherence to protocols.

Stress training courses can help people to identify the personal stressors that normally affect them, assess recent changes in those stressors, and evaluate the general level of excitement that they seek out and with which they feel comfortable. This can often be accomplished using simple paper-and-pencil exercises. Such exercises help to demonstrate the differences among squad members with respect to stressors and stress, and give each participant a chance to understand and examine his or her personal stress reactions.

Techniques for coping with stress should also be presented for discussion. In a short course or program, it is likely that only a quick overview of stress management skills can be presented. Nevertheless, the use of some simple methods can be discussed and demonstrated. It is particularly important that methods for early stress identification and stress reduction be emphasized. For example, it is valuable to know when to interrupt rescue efforts with short rest breaks. Likewise, the ability of certain foods and chemicals (such as coffee, cocoa, and tobacco) to influence stress responses should be understood. Because caffeine, sugar, and nicotine can all increase a person's response to stress, it is probably best if responders avoid them when they are under greater than usual amounts of stress at an emergency incident.

At-the-Scene Intervention

If a hazardous materials incident requires EMS responders, it probably also deserves the attention of CISD team members including peer support personnel (PSP) providers who have been trained to provide at-the-scene psychological support. PSP teams have been established in a growing number of EMS systems and communities across the country since their original development in Baltimore. When such support professionals are not currently part of existing systems, EMS and community planners should seriously consider establishing CISD programs. In smaller and nonurban communities, programs can be structured to service several neighboring systems on a shared basis. These adjunct rescuers must be knowledgeable about EMS and rescue procedures, and also be able to relate in a humanistic way to their colleagues. The qualities and abilities of particular value in these people include the following:

- Respected and trusted by their peers
- Sensitive and empathetic with others
- Familiar with stress responses, crisis intervention, and communication techniques
- Knowledgeable about emergency service procedures and operational problems in the emergency response system

Members of the PSP teams should be contacted by command officers as soon as a critical chemical exposure has been recognized and determined to warrant stress management attention. The team members should not operate as independent participants or within the inner perimeter of the contaminated zone. Their arrival and deployment should be based on strict criteria, and their activities must be directed by the incident commander (for example, the fire, medical, or security chief) who summoned them.

Team members can provide several different types of services that may be necessary for adequate psychological support at the scene. A description of these services is provided subsequently.

One-on-one counseling can be arranged for those emergency personnel who display clear and overt signs of acute stress syndromes. The need for such counseling is usually determined by team members who are assigned to observe and advise on the well-being of responders as they manage themselves and their victims. Counseling is not provided while a responder is actively involved in rescue work but only after disengagement from the operation. This "psychological watchdog'' activity provides a sort of safety net that protects rescuers from extreme, unrecognized stress and permits them to provide continuity of response services.

Advisories for incident managers can be established. This consists of advisory services that are made available to incident commanders and others with responsibilities for the safety of emergency personnel. CISD team members monitor the performance and behavior of personnel and make recommendations to the commanders about the needs of personnel and the stresses that they are encountering. For example, recommendations may involve changing duties, rotating jobs, or other adjustments of activities to relieve some rescue workers of the added stress of excessive routine or prolonged high-risk details. In other situations, recommendations may be made for brief rest periods for each responder after fixed periods of intensive rescue operations. Acceptance of such psychologically oriented advice during hazardous materials incidents can lead to decreased injuries and fatigue, less emotional stress on each responder, and higher levels of individual and group performance.

CISD team members can also contribute in an assortment of ways to *support rescuers, victims, and bystanders* to reduce disruption of essential rescue efforts. For example, interacting with response personnel during rest breaks at the emergency scene and encouraging them to speak about their experience of the incident permits release of feeling and emotions. Rescuers suffering severe stress reactions can be provided with encouragement, support, and, when necessary, removal from the scene or reassignment to lighter duty.

Postincident Management

At least two postincident stress debriefing sessions should follow hazardous materials incidents. Initially, CISD team members should be available for a short period of time immediately after the event (3 to 4 hours postincident) when responders have returned to the station or dispatch center. All rescuers should participate. This minidebriefing should be conducted by well-qualified mental health or PSP providers. The meeting is an opportunity to share information updates about long-term medical surveillance and health risks, provide support for group participation, allow ventilation of feelings, and establish the need for a more formal debriefing to follow. The typical outcome is a substantial reduction of stress responses and a more stable crew ready to go to the next emergency.

The second debriefing session is usually carried out between 1 and 3 days after the incident under the guidance of a qualified mental health provider who has participated in CISD training, or its equivalent, and who is assisted by experienced PSP team members. It is fortunate that only rarely will more than a small proportion of responders be expected to develop severe (''traumatic'') stress reactions following a critical incident. Less severe but potentially harmful stress reactions can occur in up to 80 percent of those involved. These lesser stress responses are more likely to pose a threat to health and performance if they are initially ignored.

The session involves confidential and nonevaluative group discussions about the delayed effects of stress and the actual experiences of those who participated at the emergency. The goal is to be educational. This process is not psychotherapy, but it does allow participants to understand their stress reactions, reduce the stress developing in response to the hazardous material incident, and hasten the normal recovery process.

**DEBRIEFING
PROCESS**

- Predebriefing
- Introduction
- Facts
- Thoughts
- Reactions
- Symptoms
- Teaching
- Re-entry
- Postdebriefing

Nine components to the debriefing process are as follows:

1. Predebriefing: This should be an uninterrupted session held in comfortable surroundings, possibly away from the station or dispatch center. Participants involved should not be on active duty at the time of the meeting.

2. Introduction: During this phase the MH leader explains the purpose of the session and its explicit confidentiality. All must agree to maintain confidentiality to participate. Everyone involved is given equal status and an equal voice. Criticism of another's activities is not permitted.

3. Facts: The facts of the critical incident are presented so that the entire event is recreated from a common time perspective. Discussion should not be an operational critique of actions or procedures carried out at the incident. Each participant recounts what he or she did and saw during the emergency. This may also include commenting on the roles of the PSP team members. In some cases, a participant finds that his or her story is particularly difficult to retell, or that retelling it evokes a strong emotional reaction. Others in the group can acknowledge those strong feelings, but they should not be dwelled on during the discussion.

4. Thoughts: Discussion is encouraged in which the participants recount the "first thoughts" that occurred at the moment each realized that he or she was undergoing an unusual experience and was not operating on "automatic."

5. Reactions: Participants describe the elements that were the "worst parts" of the total incident for them and how those elements made them feel. Deep psychological probing is not done. Instead, personal emotional traumas are discussed, and reassurance and support are provided.

6. Symptoms: Participants are encouraged to discuss any possible symptoms of stress that developed following the incident. Group leaders may suggest categories of symptoms, such as disturbances of sleep, memory, appetite, bowel function, and other normal functions and experiences of daily living. "How was this incident different?" is one question posed to reveal these symptoms.

7. Teaching: Based on the actual symptoms described by participants during the prior discussion, a practical guide to appropriate stress coping techniques is presented. Specific problems and techniques should be discussed.

8. Re-entry: This "wrap-up" offers additional reassurance and allows questions on any topic not covered. Follow-up activities, future changes, and preventive programs can be discussed.

9. Postdebriefing: Team members remain after the session to talk with those who have additional questions or unresolved concerns. In some cases, referrals for clinical services may be suggested. This is an important time because it acts as a bridge between the incident, the emotional ventilation of the session, and the return to normal services.

SUMMARY

Education about stress and its effects on emergency responders is becoming increasingly available and openly discussed. Additional attention needs to be paid to this area, especially because many communities cannot presently provide appropriate stress management training to emergency responders.

Like other critical incidents that demand more from rescuers than most "routine" emergency operations, hazardous materials incidents can be the source of serious psychological disability for EMS responders. Appropriate pre-incident training can encourage development of enhanced awareness and knowledge about the causes, symptoms, and reactions to stress and personal stress levels. In turn, that can contribute to improved systematic coping mechanisms. Use of established CISD teams, or their equivalent, for both at-the-scene and postincident interventions and debriefing can help to alleviate the distress that EMS responders can experience and maintain the adequacy of a community's emergency response capability.

REFERENCES

DERNOCOEUR, K., *Streetsense*. Bowie, Md.: Brady Books, 1985.

GATCHEL, R. J., and A. BAUM, *An Introduction to Health Psychology*. New York: Random House, Inc., 1983.

MITCHELL, J., and H. RESNIK, *Emergency Response to Crisis: A Crisis Intervention Guidebook for Emergency Service Personnel*. Bowie, Md.: Brady Books, 1981.

HAZARDOUS
MATERIALS DEFINITIONS

The following definitions have been abstracted from the Code of Federal Regulations, Title 49-Transportation, Parts 100 to 199. Refer to the referenced sections for complete details. *Note:* Rule-making proposals are outstanding or are contemplated concerning some of these definitions.

Hazard class	Definitions
	Explosive—Any chemical compound, mixture, or device, the primary or common purpose of which is to function by explosion, that is, with substantially instantaneous release of gas and heat, unless such compound, mixture, or device is otherwise specifically classified in Parts 170–89 (Sec. 173.50).
Class A explosive	Detonating or otherwise of maximum hazard. The nine types of class A explosives are defined in Sec. 173.53.
Class B explosive	In general, function by rapid combustion rather than detonation and include some explosive devices such as special fireworks, flash powders, and so forth. *Flammable hazard* (Sec. 173.88).
Class C explosive	Certain types of manufactured articles containing class A or B explosives, or both, as components but in restricted quantities, and certain types of fireworks. Minimum hazard (Sec. 173.100).
Blasting agents	A material designed for blasting that has been tested in accordance with Sec. 173.114a(b) and found to be so insensitive that little probability exists of accidental initiation to explosion or transition from deflagration to detonation (Sec. 173.114a[a]).
Combustible liquid	Any liquids having a flash point above 100°F and below 200°F as determined by tests listed in Sec. 173.115(d). Exceptions to this are found in Sec. 173.115(b).
Corrosive material	Any liquid or solid that causes visible destruction of human skin tissue or a liquid that has a severe corrosion rate on steel (see Sec. 173.240[a] and [b] for details). *(continued)*

APPENDIX 1 (continued):

Hazard class	Definitions
Flammable liquid	Any liquid having a flash point below 100°F as determined by tests listed in Sec. 173.115(d). Exceptions are listed in Sec. 173.115(a).
	Pyroforic liquid—Any liquid that ignites spontaneously in dry or moist air at or below 130°F (Sec. 173.115[c]).
	Compressed gas—Any material or mixture having in the container an absolute pressure exceeding 40 psia at 70°F or a pressure exceeding 104 psia at 130°F, or any liquid flammable material having a vapor pressure exceeding 40 psia at 100°F (Sec. 173.300[a]).
Flammable gas	Any compressed gas meeting the requirements for lower flammability limit, flammability limit range, flame projection, or flame propagation criteria as specified in Sec. 173.300(b).
Nonflammable gas	Any compressed gas other than a flammable compressed gas.
Flammable solid	Any solid material, other than an explosive, which is liable to cause fires through friction-retained heat from manufacturing or processing, or which can be ignited readily and when ignited burns so vigorously and persistently as to create a serious transportation hazard (Sec. 173.150).
Organic peroxide	An organic compound containing the bivalent -0-0 structure, which may be considered a derivative of hydrogen peroxide (see Sec. 173.151[a] for details).
Oxidizer	A substance such as chlorate, permanganate, inorganic peroxide, or a nitrate, that yields oxygen readily to stimulate the combustion of organic matter (Sec. 173.151).
Poison A	*Extremely dangerous poisons*—Poisonous gases or liquids of such nature that a very small amount of the gas, or vapor of the liquid, mixed with air is dangerous to life (Sec. 173.326).
Poison B	*Less dangerous poisons*—Substances, liquids, or solids (including pastes and semisolids), other than class A or irritating materials, which are known to be so toxic to humans as to afford a hazard to health during transportation; or which, in the absence of adequate data on human toxicity, are presumed to be toxic to humans (Sec. 173.343).
Irritating material	A liquid or solid substance that on contact with fire or when exposed to air gives off dangerous or intensely irritating fumes, but does not include any poisonous class A material (Sec. 173.381).
Etiologic agent	A viable micro-organism, or its toxin, which causes or may cause human disease (Sec. 173.386) (refer to the Department of Health, Education and Welfare Regulations, Title 42, CFR, 72.25[c] for details).
Radioactive material	Any material, or combination of materials, that spontaneously emits ionizing radiation, and has a specific activity greater than 0.002 μCi/g (Sec. 173.389). *Note:* See Sec. 173.389(a) through (l) for details.
	ORM-A, B, C, D or E (other regulated materials)—Any material that does not meet the definition of a hazardous material, other than a combustible liquid in packagings having a capacity of 110 gallons or less, and is specified in Sec. 172.101 as an ORM material or that possesses one or more of the characteristics described in ORM-A through D subsequently. (Sec. 173.500). *Note:* An ORM with a flash point of 100°F, when transported with more than 110 gallons in one container, shall be classed as a combustible liquid.

APPENDIX 1 (continued):

Hazard class	Definitions
ORM-A	A material that has an anesthetic, irritating, noxious, toxic, or other similar property and that can cause extreme annoyance or discomfort to passengers and crew in the event of leakage during transportation (Sec. 173.500[b][1]).
ORM-B	A material (including a solid when wet with water) capable of causing significant damage to a transport vehicle from leakage during transportation. Materials meeting one or both of the following criteria are ORM-B materials: (1) a liquid substance that has a corrosion rate exceeding 0.250 inch per year on aluminum (nonclad 7075-T6) at a test temperature of 130°F. An acceptable test is described in NACE Standard TM-01-69, and (2) specifically designated by name in Sec. 172.101 (Sec. 173.500[b][2]).
ORM-C	A material that has other inherent characteristics not described as an ORM-A or ORM-B but that make it unsuitable for shipment, unless properly identified and prepared for transportation. Each ORM-C material is specifically named in Sec. 172.101 (Sec. 173.500[b][4]).
ORM-D	A material such as a consumer commodity that presents a limited hazard during transportation because of its form, quantity, and packaging. They must be materials for which exceptions are provided in Sec. 172.101. A shipping description applicable to each ORM-D material or category of ORM-D materials is found in Sec. 172.101 (Sec. 173.500[b][4]).
ORM-E	A material that is not included in any other hazard class. Materials in this class include hazardous wastes and hazardous substances as defined in Sec. 171.8.

Additional terms used in preparation of hazardous materials for shipment (Sec. 171.8):

Consumer commodity (see ORM-D)	A material that is packaged or distributed in a form intended and suitable for sale through retail sales agencies or instrumentalities for consumption by individuals for purposes of personal care or household use. This term also includes drugs and medicines.
Flash point	The minimum temperature at which a substance gives off flammable vapors, which in contact with spark or flame will ignite (Sec. 173.115 and 173.150).
Forbidden	The hazardous material is one that must not be offered or accepted for transportation (Sec. 172.150).
Limited quantity	Means the maximum amount of hazardous material, as specified in those sections applicable to the particular hazard class. See (Sec. 173.118, 173.118[a], 173.153, 173.244, 173.306, 173.345 and 173.364).
Spontaneously combustible material (solid)	A solid substance (including sludges and pastes) that may undergo spontaneous heating or self-ignition under conditions normally incident to transportation or that may undergo an increase in temperature and ignite on contact with the atmosphere.
Water-reactive material (solid)	Any solid substance (including sludges and pastes) that, by interaction with water, is likely to become spontaneously flammable or give off flammable or toxic gases in dangerous quantities.

COMMAND SYSTEMS

Many hazardous materials incidents involve several separate emergency response services and personnel. For example, a motor vehicle accident involving a tanker truck could easily result in responses by fire service, police, EMS, hazardous materials teams, environmental protection services, transportation specialists, and others. Coordinating these various teams and their personnel to effect an optimal response and assure the safety of all the responders can pose a complex and difficult task.

For this reason, part of the preplanning for hazardous materials incidents should involve the development of a clear and orderly command system. Such a system must allow for the coordination of all possible response groups and their different functions and personnel assignments. It must also anticipate the likely presence of news media representatives and spectators at every incident.

The goal of that command system is to create a uniform approach for command operations and situation evaluation. No single best system exists. In every region, a system should be developed that considers the actual needs and resources available in that area.

PERSON IN CHARGE

To maintain the safety and orderly function of a hazardous materials operation, a need exists for a clear line of command. Response personnel should never have to ask "Who's in charge?"

Generally, the first arriving fire officer becomes the officer in charge (OIC) at the incident. This person should be clearly identified as the incident commander. The incident communications center and all emergency personnel should be informed of his or her identity and role.

The OIC must then establish an explicit management system for the incident, which involves several related functions.

1. Determine the goals and objectives of the response operations.
2. Set up a command post and assure that all personnel know where it is located.
3. Determine the level of response needed to achieve the goals and objectives, and request the assistance necessary.
4. Establish a staging area in a safe place for arriving personnel and equipment. Separate staging areas for EMS and medical supplies may be necessary at large incidents.

The OIC must be ready to turn over command when a more senior or more qualified officer arrives and is willing to assume command.

COMMAND POST

The command post should be conspicuous and, it is hoped, located in a safe location. The components of that post will depend in part on the size and needs of the incident and in part on the actual equipment and materials readily available. A protected, indoor work area with desks, lighting, reference materials, communication equipment, and space should be available for staff. In sophisticated organizations, an all-weather vehicle housing computers and other office equipment may be used as mobile command posts.

The most important function of the command post is to allow the OIC and his or her advisors a protected place to consult, plan, and organize the response.

SECTORS: DELEGATION AND DIVISION OF COMMAND

It is useful to divide the tactical response to a hazardous materials incident into manageable component functions. The OIC can then assign each component function to a different person who becomes responsible for commanding that component operation. These component functions are commonly referred to as *sectors*. The OIC should divide the response into sectors and assign them as quickly as possible once the response has begun.

The persons assigned sector command responsibilities are known as *sector officers*. They are usually chosen because of their experience and seniority. Like the OIC, these persons should be clearly identified, and all emergency responders under their command should be aware of their role. Sector officers are responsible for carrying out their sector, protecting the responders under their command, and reporting regularly to the OIC.

Only a few or a great many sectors may be at an incident. The number will usually be determined by the nature and size of the incident and the resources available to the OIC. A list of possible sectors at a large incident would include the following:

1. *Emergency medical services:* Coordinates all medical and health concerns at the incident.
2. *Hazard:* Oversees the actual management of the response to the hazardous material that has provoked the incident. This sector includes the hot and warm zones, and the most immediate dangers at the incident. It is often further divided into component subsectors.
3. *Safety:* Monitors the incident and personnel, assures compliance with safety procedures, limits access to hot and warm zones of incident.
4. *Staging:* Controls and oversees equipment and personnel inventories.
5. *Police:* Coordinates interaction between law enforcement personnel and emergency response operations.
6. *Public information:* Provides information to media.
7. *Resources:* Assures adequate numbers of personnel and equipment to the operating sectors of the response.
8. *Rehabilitation:* Provides food, liquids, and medical supervision of operating personnel in a safe, clean location.

CONFINEMENT
AND CONTAINMENT

Confinement and containment name two types of techniques by which emergency responders can limit or influence the spread and distribution of a leaking hazardous material. It is not likely that EMS responders will be asked to carry out these tasks, but all responders at a hazardous materials incident should understand how and why they are performed.

CONFINEMENT

Confinement activities are intended to control the spread of a hazardous material. They are defensive techniques that can be carried out at a safe distance from the leaking hazard. Because confinement techniques require relatively simple tools and equipment, they can be readily carried out by first responders. These techniques can be grouped into three separate categories: diversion, diking, and retention.

Diversion is used to direct the flow of a spilled liquid to an area where it will produce less damage and harm. This is generally accomplished by building a low barrier that diverts the flowing stream and controls its movement. A diversion barrier might be used, for example, to direct the flow of fuel oil or other flammable liquids away from storm drains and sewer systems.

Diversion barriers should be constructed far ahead of the flowing material so that the barrier can be completed before the flow arrives. They are useful as the first and simplest form of control available to emergency responders.

Dikes are a means of containing hazardous materials and preventing their flow to areas where they can cause greater harm. The dikes form temporary containment areas that hold the materials. Diking is useful as a temporary solution to be used while more permanent solutions are being developed.

Dikes can be built out of dirt or heavy materials that are found at the inci-

259

dent site. Pieces of wood, tree limbs, boards, and sand bags are other examples. Once constructed, the dikes can be draped by plastic tarps or salvage covers. For large leaks, diking may require construction equipment and truck loads of materials.

Retention techniques are used to close off storm drains and sewer systems to prevent hazardous materials from flowing into them. Those drains, for example, can be blocked by plastic tarps or salvage covers that are then covered by a layer of dirt or sand. The retention area thus created allows liquid hazardous materials to form a pool on top of the retention barrier rather than enter the sewer drain.

CONTAINMENT

Containment activities are intended to control a hazardous material leak and keep that material within its container. They are offensive techniques that must be carried out in the hot zone. Containment techniques usually require special tools and equipment, more extensive personal protective equipment, and decontamination of the entry team members after they have performed the activities.

Because of the increased risk associated with containment activities, they should not be initiated before a risk evaluation of the incident has been completed. The OIC must determine that the appropriate equipment and personal protective equipment are available, the entry team has the skills required to perform the necessary activities, and decontamination and emergency care are prepared for the entry team.

The risks of containment activities are justified when defensive confinement activities have not been successful, and a substantial likelihood exists that leaking hazardous materials will be dispersed and cause harm to the environment or surrounding communities. The benefits of a successful containment activity include minimized environmental damage, limited dispersion of hazards, reduced operating time, and decreased cleanup needs.

Containment activities should only be carried out by responders who have received specific training in the skills and techniques required. Such techniques include the following:

1. Use of plugs and patches for containers

2. Reduction of pressure in pressurized containers

3. Application of vapor suppression agents

4. Chemical neutralization

5. Absorption and disposal

MEDICAL SURVEILLANCE

Medical surveillance names the health monitoring program that is required by the OSHA to protect the health and safety of workers who are at risk of exposure to hazardous chemicals. The goal of this program is to assure that workers exposed to hazardous materials are monitored so that they do not develop chronic diseases, disability, or death as a result of overexposure. For workers routinely exposed to hazardous materials, another goal is to assure that they are healthy and can safely use personal protective equipment.

For their own protection, emergency response personnel and others who may work with hazardous materials should make themselves aware of these requirements. The OSHA requirements are contained in a set of regulations called the Hazardous Waste Operations and Emergency Response Standard (29 *Code of Federal Regulations* 1910.120). This standard addresses the following two groups of workers:

1. Many hazardous waste site workers and members of hazardous materials teams

2. Emergency response personnel

The requirements for medical surveillance are different for these two groups. Hazardous waste site workers and hazardous materials team members must undergo more extensive medical surveillance than emergency responders. Most EMS and other medical personnel will be regarded as emergency response personnel and will receive less extensive medical surveillance.

Medical surveillance involves periodic medical examinations and consultations. Those examinations and consultations must be made available at the expense of the employer. They should be performed by a licensed physician, preferably one knowledgeable in occupational medicine. The contents of the examination or consultations are determined by that physician and may include laboratory testing. The employer should give the worker a copy of the physician's findings, recommendations, and test results.

For hazardous waste site workers and members of hazardous materials teams, medical surveillance examinations should be performed according to the following schedule:

1. Prior to assignment (pre-employment screening)

2. At least every 12 months unless the attending physician believes a longer time interval (up to 24 months) is more appropriate

3. At termination of employment or reassignment to a job without exposure if the last medical surveillance examination was more than 6 months earlier

4. As soon as possible if a worker develops signs or symptoms of possible overexposure

5. As soon as possible if a worker suffers exposure above the permissible exposure limit without the necessary personal protective equipment at an emergency

For emergency responders, medical surveillance examinations are not routinely provided. They must be provided, however, under the following circumstances:

1. As soon as possible if an emergency responder develops signs or symptoms of possible overexposure as a result of an exposure to hazardous materials at an emergency incident

2. As soon as possible if an emergency responder suffers exposure above the permissible exposure limit without the necessary personal protective equipment at an emergency incident

3. At additional times if the attending physician determines that follow-up examinations or consultations are necessary

Members of volunteer services are not necessarily covered by these regulations. Each state has the right to determine whether volunteers are regarded as "employees" and, therefore, covered. Members of volunteer emergency response services should determine how they are to be treated in their own states.

REQUIRED HAZARDOUS MATERIALS TRAINING FOR EMS PERSONNEL

APPENDIX 5

Concern about the harmful effects of hazardous materials accidents has led to public demand for greater levels of emergency preparedness. In the United States, several federal and state laws have been enacted to address those concerns. Examples of such laws include Title III of the SARA, and related regulations developed by the EPA and OSHA.

One important goal of those laws and regulations is to enhance the skills and knowledge of emergency response personnel who might be called to hazardous materials incidents. Another goal is to protect the health and safety of those emergency responders. To accomplish both goals, emergency response training has been required for many response personnel.

SARA Title III, for example, requires the development of local emergency response plans that must include "Training programs, including schedules for training of local emergency response and medical personnel."[1] Submission of local emergency response plans was required by October 1988. In theory, therefore, training programs required under SARA should have been scheduled by that time. The actual informational content to be included in such training programs was not clearly stated in SARA.

More comprehensive and explicit demands for training and other safety programs were published by OSHA in 1989. Those demands are found in the Hazardous Waste Operations and Emergency Response Standard, also known as 29 *CFR* 1910.120, which regulates "the safety and health of employees in . . . any emergency response to incidents involving hazardous substances."[2]

Under that OSHA standard, training is required for all employees "who participate, or are expected to participate, in emergency response to hazardous substance accidents."[3] OSHA lists many emergency responders, including EMS personnel, among those who must be trained: "Emergency response personnel include firefighters, EMS personnel, and police as well as other employees."[4] According to OSHA, the actual training should be tailored to fit the work that individuals are expected to carry out: "Training shall be based on the duties and function to be performed by each responder of an emergency response organization."[5]

OSHA'S TIERED TRAINING SCHEME

Explicit descriptions of the training required for most emergency responders is contained in the OSHA standard. A tiered training scheme is presented with four training levels that correspond to four different levels of emergency response skills.[6] Each skills level corresponds to a substantially different role during an incident.

1. First-responder awareness
2. First-responder operations
3. Hazardous materials technician
4. Hazardous materials specialist

Unfortunately, the OSHA standard does not correlate those training levels to EMS performance skills. Likewise, it does not indicate the appropriate performance level for EMS responders. As a result, no clear indication is given of the amount of training that EMS personnel should receive.

EMS personnel might be asked to perform at any of the first three performance levels. The circumstances of an emergency and the response protocols of the specific EMS service will determine their actual level of performance. Accordingly, EMS training needs can vary widely. EMS system supervisors should determine guidelines and protocols for EMS response to hazardous materials incidents to determine the scope of needed training.

First-responder awareness.   Under some circumstances, EMS personnel might be expected to function at the first-responder awareness level. According to OSHA, those are persons

> who are likely to witness or discover a hazardous substance release and who have been trained to initiate an emergency response sequence by notifying the proper authorities of the release. They would take no further action beyond notifying the authorities.[7]

EMS personnel operating at this level would not be expected actually to perform EMS skills at hazardous materials incidents. Instead of caring for incident victims, their functions would be restricted to observing and reporting. An EMS system probably could not provide care to exposure victims if all of its personnel were trained to only this performance level.

OSHA expects training for the first-responder awareness level to provide competency in the following areas:

1. Understanding of what hazardous materials are and the risks associated with them

2. Understanding of the potential outcomes associated with a hazardous materials emergency

3. Ability to recognize the presence of hazardous materials in an emergency

4. Ability to identify hazardous materials, if possible

5. Understanding of role of first-responder awareness person including site security and control, and use of the DOT's *Emergency Response Guidebook*

6. Ability to realize the need for additional resources

First-responder operations. It is more likely that EMS personnel would function at the first-responder operations level. As described by OSHA, these persons

> respond to releases or potential releases of hazardous substances as part of the initial response to the site for the purpose of protecting nearby persons, property, or the environment from the effects of the release. They are trained to respond in a defensive fashion without actually trying to stop the release. Their function is to contain the release from a safe distance, keep it from spreading, and prevent exposures.[8]

This role description could include EMS functions. As written, however, it more specifically describes the functions of fire service personnel and other non-EMS hazardous materials response team members. Responders at this performance level are expected to work at a "safe distance" from the incident. Hence, this performance level is below that of EMS personnel who might enter contaminated places to perform clinical assessment or management, rapid extrication, or decontamination of heavily exposed victims.

Training for the first-responder operations level entails at least 8 hours and should provide students with competency in the following areas in addition to those listed for the awareness level:

1. Knowledge of basic hazard and risk assessment techniques

2. Ability to select and use proper personal protective equipment

3. Understanding of basic hazardous materials terms

4. Ability to perform basic control, containment, and confinement within the limits of equipment and resources available to the response unit

5. Knowledge of basic decontamination procedures

6. Understanding of relevant standard operating procedures

It is unclear whether OSHA regards EMS medical protocols for the care of exposure victims as a type of hazardous materials "standard operating procedure." It is logical to consider such protocols as equivalent to standard operating procedures. EMS hazardous materials training should emphasize EMS and medical protocols that relate to the clinical care of exposure victims. The amount of training time devoted to such protocols will necessarily vary according to the extent and complexity of a system's protocols.

Another uncertainty in the OSHA regulations concerns control, containment, and confinement. It is not clear how extensively EMS personnel should be trained in these skills, because most EMS personnel are unlikely to perform them. One approach is to explain briefly the role and purpose of control, containment, and confinement without teaching them as performance skills.

Hazardous materials technician.   These individuals "approach the point of release in order to plug, patch or otherwise stop the release of a hazardous substance."[9] The functions that they perform, as described in 29 *CFR* 1910.120, are clearly different from those of EMS personnel. It is not difficult, however, to imagine situations in which EMS personnel might "approach the point of release" by entering contaminated places to provide on-scene care or assessment, rapid extrication, or decontamination of heavily contaminated victims. In such situations, EMS responders share many of the risks experienced by fire service hazardous materials technicians. These EMS responders would benefit from the theoretical and self-protective information provided at this performance level. It is unclear, however, whether OSHA intended EMS personnel to be trained at this level.

Training for the hazardous materials technician level entails at least 24 hours. Training should provide students with competency in the following areas in addition to those listed for the first-responder awareness and operations levels:

1. Understanding of the employer's emergency response plan

2. Ability to use detection instruments to identify and verify known and unknown hazardous materials

3. Ability to function within an assigned role in the incident command system

4. Ability to select and use proper specialized chemical personal protective equipment

5. Understanding of hazard and risk assessment techniques

6. Ability to perform advanced control, containment, and confinement operations within the limits of equipment and resources available to the response unit

7. Understanding and ability to implement decontamination

8. Understanding of termination procedures

9. Understanding of basic chemical and toxicologic terminology

Hazardous materials specialist. Some emergency responders are expected to provide support and advanced knowledge to hazardous materials technicians. They may also be called on to act as liaison with Federal, state and local authorities in regards to site activities. Such responders, known as hazardous materials specialists, also have duties that parallel those of hazardous materials technicians. It is unlikely that EMS personnel will be expected to operate at this level.

Hazardous materials specialists should receive at least 24 hours of training equal to the technician level. In addition, OSHA expects these responders to have the following competency:

1. Know how to implement the local emergency response plan

2. Understand use of advanced survey instruments and equipment

3. Know state emergency response plan

4. Understand in-depth hazard and risk techniques

5. Ability to determine and implement decontamination procedures

6. Ability to perform specialized control, containment and confinement operations

7. Ability to develop a site safety and control plan

8. Understand chemical, radiological, and toxicological terminology and behavior

TRAINER QUALIFICATIONS

To provide training to EMS personnel satisfactorily, communities and EMS systems will need competent trainers. Because much of the material included in an EMS training program on hazardous materials goes beyond standard EMS teaching, instructors will need to be selected on the basis of advanced training or specialized skills.

The importance of such skilled faculty is stressed by the OSHA in 29 *CFR* 1910.120.

Trainers . . . shall have satisfactorily completed a training course for teaching the subjects they are expected to teach, such as the courses offered by the U.S. Fire Academy, or they shall have the training and/or academic credentials and instructional experience necessary to demonstrate competent instructional skills and a good command of the subject matter of the courses they are to teach.[10]

CERTIFICATION

The OSHA allows two ways to satisfy its standard. One way, as described earlier, involves systematic training of emergency responders. The other permits an emergency responder to demonstrate competency in those skills that are appropriate to his or her performance level. If a person can objectively demonstrate competency, then training is not required.

"The employer shall so certify" that the standard has been satisfied by either a training program or by demonstration of competency.[11] If a statement of competency is made by an employer, then a record must be kept of the methods by which competency was demonstrated.

In addition, emergency responders must receive retraining annually that is "of sufficient content and duration to maintain their competencies."[12] Alternatively, employees can be asked to demonstrate competency at least yearly. The employer should certify that competency has been demonstrated or that adequate training has been provided to the emergency responder employee.

1. Superfund Amendments and Reauthorization Act of 1986, Title III, §303(c) (8), 100 *STAT* 1732.
2. *Federal Register,* 54 (March 6, 1989), 9294.
3. Ibid., 9298–99.
4. Ibid., 9300.
5. Ibid., 9329.
6. Ibid., 9310, 9329.
7. Ibid., 9329.
8. Ibid., 9329.
9. Ibid., 9329.
10. Ibid., 9330.
11. Ibid., 9329–90.
12. Ibid., 9330.

GLOSSARY

Absorption. Absorption refers to the taking up of liquids into the body. Absorption also describes the process by which liquid hazardous materials are soaked up to limit the spread of contamination.

Accident. An unexpected event generally resulting in injury, loss of property, or disruption of service.

ACGIH. American Conference of Governmental Industrial Hygienists.

Acute exposure. A dose that is delivered to the body in a single event or in a short period.

Air purification devices. Respirators or filtration devices that remove particulate matter, gases, or vapors from the atmosphere. These devices range from full-face–piece, dual-cartridge masks with eye protection to half-mask, face-piece–mounted cartridges with no eye protection.

Air-reactive materials. Substances with low autoignition temperatures.

Air supply devices. Respirators that provide compressed air, at pressures that are greater than atmospheric pressure, to a face mask that is worn by a rescuer.

Airways. The routes for passage of air from the nose and mouth to the alveolar sacs of the lungs.

Alkali. A basic compound that has the ability to neutralize an acid and form a salt.

Alveolar ducts. The smallest of the lungs' airways that connect terminal bronchioles and alveolar sacs. Sometimes called respiratory bronchioles.

269

Alveoli. Microscopic air sacs of the lungs where gas exchange occurs with the circulatory system.

Anoxia. Absence or lack of oxygen.

Anterior chamber. The fluid-filled anterior portion of the eye that rests between the cornea and the lens.

Apnea. Temporary suspension of breathing.

Asphyxia. A condition in which cells are deprived of oxygen.

Assessment. Evaluation of the condition of a patient.

Asthma. Constriction of the bronchial tubes, in response to irritation, allergy, or other stimulus.

Autoignition temperature. The lowest temperature at which a flammable gas or vapor-air mixture will ignite from its own heat source or a contacted heated surface without necessity of spark or flame.

Battle's sign. Swelling and discoloration behind the ear caused by a fracture of the base of the skull.

Boiling point. The temperature at which liquid changes its phase to a vapor or gas; the temperature at which the pressure of the liquid equals atmospheric pressure.

Breakthrough time. The elapsed time between the application of a chemical to a protective material's outer surface and its initial appearance at the inner surface.

Breach. An opening in a hazardous materials container through which hazardous material matter can escape.

Bronchi. The larger air passages within the lungs.

Bronchioles. The finer subdivisions of the branched bronchial tree.

Bronchitis. Inflammation of the bronchial tubes.

Bronchospasm. Contraction of the smooth muscle of the bronchi.

Catecholamines. Substances produced by the nervous system such as epinephrine (adrenaline) and dopamine, which increase the heart rate and blood pressure.

Caustic. Substance that strongly irritates, burns, corrodes, or destroys living tissue.

CERCLA. The Comprehensive Environmental Response Compensation and Liability Act of 1980, also known as Superfund.

Chemical degradation. The altering of the chemical structure of a hazardous material during the process of decontamination.

Chemical protective clothing. Clothing specifically designed to protect the skin and eyes from direct chemical contact. The two types are nonencapsulating and encapsulating.

Chemical resistance. The ability of chemical protective clothing to maintain its integrity and protection qualities when it comes into contact with a hazardous material.

Chronic exposure. Low doses repeatedly received by the body during a long period of time.

Cilia. Tiny hairlike ''whips'' on the surface of the bronchi and other respiratory passages that aid in the removal of mucus and particulate matter from the airways.

Coagulation necrosis. The destructive process by which acids cause proteins to precipitate as a dense, clotlike ''coagulum'' that covers the injured area.

Collagen. A protein that is the main supportive protein of skin, cornea, tendon, bone, and connective tissue.

Colorimetric tubes. Devices that are used to determine the presence and approximate concentration of chemicals that might be found in the atmosphere to be tested.

Combustible gas indicators. Devices that measure the air concentration of a flammable gas or vapor for which the indicator has been specifically calibrated.

Combustible liquid. Any liquid that has a flash point at or above 100°F (37.7°C) and below 200°F (93.3°C).

Compatibility chart. A chart that rates the strength of a protective clothing material against exposure to specified chemicals.

Conducting airways. The largest of the airway tubes. They include the trachea, bronchi, and larger bronchioles.

Confinement. Those procedures taken to keep a material in a defined or local area.

Conjunctiva. The delicate mucous membrane that lines the eyelids and covers the exposed surface of the eyeball.

Contact dermatitis. The inflammatory skin reaction caused by a skin irritant.

Containment. Those procedures taken to keep a material in its container.

Contaminant/contamination.   A substance or process that poses a threat to life, health, or the environment.

Control.   The procedures, techniques, and methods used in the mitigation of a hazardous materials incident.

Control zone.   The designation of areas at a hazardous materials incident based on safety and the degree of hazard. Will generally include the hot (exclusion) zone, the warm (decontamination) zone, and the clean (support) zone.

Contusion.   Bruising; the reaction of soft tissue to a direct blow.

Cornea.   Transparent membrane covering the anterior portion of the eye.

Corneal stroma.   The connective tissue that constitutes the middle of the cornea. The stroma, which accounts for most corneal tissue, is primarily made of collagen and mucopolysaccharides.

Corneum stratum.   Superficial membrane of dead, dried cells overlying the epidermis.

Corrosion.   The destruction of the texture or substance of a tissue.

Corrosives.   Substances that destroy the texture or substance of tissues.

Cryogenics.   The field of science dealing with the behavior of matter at low temperatures.

Debriefing.   A postincident review that primarily focuses on the adequacy of response plans and needs for systematic changes.

Decontamination.   The physical or chemical process of removing hazardous materials from exposed persons and equipment at a hazardous materials incident.

Degradation.   A chemical action involving the molecular breakdown of a protective clothing material because of contact with a chemical. Degradation is noted by visible signs such as charring, shrinking, or dissolving, or by testing the clothing material for weight changes, loss of fabric tensile strength, and so forth.

Dermis.   The inner layer of the skin, found beneath the epidermis. This layer is rich in blood vessels, nerves, and skin structures.

Desiccation.   Violent mechanical dehydration of cells.

Dike.   A barrier that prevents passage of a hazardous material to an area where it will produce more harm.

Dilution.   The use of water to flush a hazardous material from protective clothing and equipment.

Direct-acting chemicals. Chemicals that are able to cause harm without first being transformed or changed.

Direct-reading instrument. A portable device that measures and displays in a short time the concentration of a contaminant in the environment.

Diversion. Controlled movement of a hazardous material to an area where it will produce less harm.

DOT. The U.S. Department of Transportation; the federal agency that regulates the transportation of hazardous materials; also publishes aids for emergency response.

DOT hazard classifications. The hazard class designations for specific hazardous materials as found in DOT regulations.

Durability. The ability of chemical protective clothing to resist tearing and punctures.

Dyspnea. Difficult or labored breathing.

Emergency. A sudden and unexpected event calling for immediate remedial action.

Environmental emergencies. Incidents involving the release (or potential release) of hazardous materials into the environment that require immediate corrective action.

Environmental hazard. A condition capable of posing an unreasonable risk to air, water, or soil quality, and to plants or wildlife.

Enzyme poisons. Chemicals that inhibit specific cellular reactions by competing with or altering the enzymes necessary to catalyze those reactions.

Epidermis. The outermost and nonvascular layer of the skin.

Evacuation. A prolonged precautionary stay away from an area affected by a hazardous material.

Exothermic reactions. Chemical reactions that produce heat.

Expansion ratio. The volume of gas produced by the vaporization of a given volume of liquid.

Explosives. Compounds that are unstable and break down with the sudden release of large amounts of energy.

Extrication. Any actions that disentangle and free from entrapment.

First responder. The first trained personnel to arrive on the scene of a hazardous materials incident—usually officials from local emergency services, firefighters, and police.

Flammability.   The capacity of a substance to ignite and burn rapidly.

Flammable (explosive) range.   The range of gas or vapor concentration (percentage by volume in air) that will burn or explode if an ignition source is present. Limiting concentrations are commonly called the *lower explosive limit* and the *upper explosive limit*. Below the flammable limit the mixture is too lean to burn; above the upper flammable limit the mixture is too rich to burn.

Flash point.   The minimum temperature at which a liquid gives off enough vapors to ignite and flash over, but not continue to burn without the addition of more heat.

Flexibility.   Elasticity. Determines the ease with which a responder can work while wearing chemical protective clothing.

Fumes.   Fine particles of dust dispersed in air.

Gases.   A state of matter in which the material has low density and viscosity; can expand and contract greatly in response to changes in temperature and pressure; easily diffuses into other gases; readily and uniformly distributes itself throughout any container.

Hazard.   A circumstance or condition that can cause harm.

Hazardous.   Capable of posing an unreasonable risk to health and safety (DOT definition). Capable of doing harm.

Hazardous materials.   Any substance which jumps out of its container when something goes wrong, and hurts or harms the things it touches (Benner definition).

Hazardous substance.   Generally, a hazardous material. Specifically, this term has been defined for regulatory purposes in the United States: (1) A material and its mixtures or solutions that is identified by the letter "E" in the first column of the Hazardous Materials Table, 49 CFR 172.101, when offered for transportation in one package, or in one transport vehicle if not packaged, and when the quantity of the material therein equals or exceeds the reportable quantity. (2) Any substance designated pursuant to Section 311(b)(2) (a) of the Federal Water Pollution Control Act; (b) any element, compound, mixture, solution, or substance designated pursuant to Section 102 of this act; (c) any hazardous waste having the characteristics identified under or listed pursuant to Section 3001 of the Solid Waste Disposal Act (but not including any waste that, the regulation of which under the Solid Waste Disposal Act, has been suspended by an act of Congress; (d) any toxic pollutant listed under Section 307(a) of the Federal Water Pollution Control Act; (e) any hazardous air pollutant listed under Section 112 of the Clean Air Act; and (f) any imminently hazardous chemical substance or mixture with respect to which the administrator has taken action pursuant to Section 7 of the Toxic Substances Control Act. The term does not include petroleum, including crude oil or any fraction thereof that is not otherwise specifically listed or designated as a hazardous substance under subparagraphs (a) through (f) of this paragraph and the term does not include natural gas, natural gas liquids, liquified natural gas, or synthetic gas usable for fuel (of mixtures of natural gas and such synthetic gas).

Hazardous materials incident.   The release or potential release of a hazardous material from its container into the environment.

Hemolysis.   Sudden, acute destruction of red blood cells.

Hypergolic materials.   Materials that ignite spontaneously on contact with one another without requiring a source of ignition.

Hypocalcemia.   Reduction of the blood calcium below normal.

Ignition (autoignition) temperature.   The minimum temperature required to ignite gas or vapor without a spark or flame being present.

IDLH.   Immediately dangerous to life and health.

Immediately dangerous to life and health (IDLH).   That atmospheric concentration of a chemical that poses an immediate danger to the life or health of a person who is exposed but from which that person could escape without any escape-impairing symptoms or irreversible health effects. A companion measurement to the permissible exposure limit, IDLH concentrations represent levels at which respiratory protection is required. IDLH is expressed in parts per million (ppm) or mg/cu meter.

Incident.   The release or potential release of a hazardous substance into the environment.

Incident commander.   The person responsible for establishing and managing the overall operational plan. This process includes developing an effective organizational structure, allocating resources, making appropriate assignments, managing information, and continually attempting to achieve the basic command objectives.

Indirect-acting chemicals.   Chemicals that must be transformed before they can provoke injury.

Insecticide.   A poison that is used to kill insects.

Iris.   The circular pigmented membrane behind the cornea, perforated by the pupil.

Ischemia.   Lack of blood supply to a part of the body leading to lack of oxygen and other blood-borne nutrients.

Ischemic necrosis.   Death of cells as a result of lack of blood flow to the affected tissues.

Laryngitis.   Inflammation of the larynx.

Laryngospasm.   Spasmodic closure of the larynx.

LEL.   Lower explosive limit. Below the lower explosive limit not enough vapor is present for a chemical to burn.

Liquefaction necrosis.   The destructive process by which alkali cause cell death and turn solid tissue into a soapy liquid.

mg/cu meter.   Milligrams per cubic meter of air.

Mitigation.   Actions taken to prevent or reduce the severity of harm.

Mists.   Liquid droplets dispersed in air.

MSDS.   Material safety data sheet. Used throughout industry as a means of identifying chemicals.

Mucopolysaccharides.   Complex sugars that are found throughout the body and in many organs as an important component of connective tissue. These sugars may be attached to proteins. When dissolved in water, they form mucin.

Nasopharynx.   The part of the pharynx that lies above the level of the soft palate.

Necrosis.   Death of tissue, usually as individual cells, groups of cells, or in small localized areas.

NIOSH.   National Institute for Occupational Safety and Health.

Ocular.   Pertaining to the eye.

Opacified.   Having become opaque.

OSHA.   Occupational Safety and Health Administration.

Oxygen meters.   Devices that measure the proportion of oxygen in the surrounding atmosphere.

Palpation.   Examination by touch.

PEL.   Permissible exposure limit.

Permissible exposure limit.   The maximum average concentration (averaged over 8 continuous hours) to which 95 percent of otherwise healthy adults can be repeatedly and safely exposed for periods of 8 hours per day, 40 hours per week.

Penetration.   The movement of material through a suit's closures, such as zippers, buttonholes, seams, flaps, or other design features.

Percutaneous absorption.   Skin absorption of chemicals.

Permeation. A chemical action involving the movement of chemicals, on a molecular level, through intact material.

Permeation rate. A measure of the quantity of chemical that permeates a given area of material in a given time.

pH. A measure of a substance's ability to react as an acid (low pH) or as an alkali (high pH).

Polymer. Any of numerous natural and synthetic compounds of usually high molecular weight consisting of up to millions of repeated linked units, each a relatively light and simple molecule.

ppm. Parts per million.

Pulmonary edema. Collection of extravascular fluid in the lungs, usually owing either to increased intravascular pressure or increased permeability of the pulmonary capillaries. Edema fluid can impair breathing by making the lung tissues heavy and by filling alveolar sacs with fluids.

Pupil. The opening at the center of the iris of the eye for transmission of light.

Raccoon eyes. Swelling and discoloration around both eyes; a late sign of basilar skull fracture.

Radiation meters. Devices that detect the presence and measure the quantity of radiation emitted by the decay of radioactive substances.

Reactivity. The ability of a substance to interact with other substances and body tissues.

Respiratory bronchioles. The smallest of the airway tubules. They connect the larger bronchioles to the alveoli. Sometimes called alveolar ducts.

Routes of exposure. The manner in which a chemical contaminant enters the body.

SARA. The Superfund Amendments and Reauthorization Act of 1986.

SCBA. Self-contained breathing apparatus.

Sclera. The tough white supporting tunic of the eyeball.

Sequestration agents. Agents that bind specific salts and make them unavailable to the cells.

Sloughing. The process by which necrotic cells separate from the tissues to which they have been attached. Airway cells, for example, can slough and fall into the bronchiolar lumen, or corneal epithelial cells may slough and slide away from the cornea.

Solubility. The ability of a solid, liquid, gas, or vapor to dissolve in a solvent; the ability of one material to blend uniformly with another.

Solvent. A liquid substance capable of dissolving another substance.

Specific gravity. The ratio of the mass of a unit volume of a substance to the mass of the same volume of a standard substance at a standard temperature.

Stridor. A harsh, high-pitched respiratory sound such as the inspiratory sound often heard in acute laryngeal obstruction.

Surfactant. A surface-active agent that plays an important role in keeping alveoli functional.

Symblepharon. An adhesion between the two surfaces of the conjunctivae, usually formed during the healing of a burn, that restricts the ability of the lid to open and close.

Thromboses. Formation of a blood clot in a blood vessel or within a chamber of the heart.

TLV-C. Threshold limit value-ceiling.

Threshold limit value-ceiling. The maximum concentration to which a healthy adult can be exposed without risk of injury.

TLV–STEL. Threshold limit value–short-term exposure limit.

Threshold limit value–short-term exposure limit. The maximum average concentration (averaged over a continuous 15-minute period) to which an otherwise healthy adult can be safely exposed for up to 15 minutes continuously.

TLV–TWA. Threshold limit value–time-weighted average.

Threshold limit value–time-weighted average. The maximum average concentration (averaged over 8 continuous hours) to which an otherwise healthy adult can be repeatedly and safely exposed for periods of 8 hours per day, 40 hours per week.

Toxicity. The ability of a substance to produce injury once it reaches a susceptible site in or on the body.

Tracheitis. Inflammation of the trachea.

UEL. Upper explosive limit. Above the upper explosive limit the mixture of air and vapor is too rich for a chemical to burn.

Unstable monomers. Highly reactive chemicals that are normally used in the production of synthetic fibers and plastics.

Vapor density. The weight of a given volume of vapor or gas compared to the weight of an equal volume of dry air, both measured at the same temperature and pressure.

Vapor pressure.   A measure of the tendency of a liquid to vaporize into a gas.

Vapors.   The gaseous form of substances that are normally in the solid or liquid state at room temperature and pressure.

Vascular.   Pertaining to the blood vessels.

Vesiculation.   The presence or formation of vesicles (blisters).

Water-reactive materials.   Any substance that readily reacts with or decomposes in the presence of water with substantial energy release.

Water solubility.   The quantity of a chemical that will mix or dissolve in water.

Wheezing.   Whistling sounds made in breathing; a sign of spasm or narrowing of the bronchi.

INDEX

A

Acetone, 16, 27

Acids:
  and reactivity, 27, 197
  antidotes, 170
  coagulation necrosis, 115
  decontamination, 143, 145, 146
  detection of, 75
  exposure to, 110, 111, 112, 113, 114,
      115, 123, 162, 198, 200, 201, 203,
      208, 210-13, 214, 220, 223-25, 228
  protection from, 92, 100, 157, 184
  removal and treatment of, 80, 212-13,
      226-27
Agency for Toxic Substances and Dis-
      ease Registry (ATSDR), 69
Agricultural chemicals:
  herbicides, 45
  insecticides, 4, 45, 100, 126, 156, 158,
      164, 165, 167, 238-39, 195-97,
      295, 300-302
  pesticides, 45, 238
  warning systems, 45
Air purification devices, 85-86, 91, 100
Air-reactive chemicals, 27, 28
Air supply devices, 85, 87-88, 100

Airway assessment, 119
Airway management, 155-57, 167, 200
  cricothyroidotomy, 156
  nasopharyngeal airway, 155, 156
  oropharyngeal airway, 155, 156
Airway obstruction, 19, 121, 155, 156,
      200
Alkali, 28, 75, 78-80, 92, 100, 111, 113,
      114, 115, 123, 143, 145, 146, 157,
      162-63, 164, 166, 184, 197, 200,
      201, 203, 208, 210-15, 216, 217,
      220, 223, 224, 225, 226, 227, 230
Alkylating agents, 28, 115, 199, 208, 217,
      224
Allergic reactions, 158, 161, 198, 201,
      220, 223
Aluminum alkyls:
  pyrophoric materials, 31
American Council of Governmental and
      Industrial Hygienists (ACGIH),
      30, 31, 32
Ammonia, 4, 5, 40, 85, 110, 111, 114, 121,
      156, 157, 197, 200, 210, 222, 225
Anesthetics, 121, 160-61, 170
Antidotes, 107, 131, 167-71, 236
Arsine, 126, 236
Asphyxiants, 121, 158, 165-66, 235-37
Assessment, 105, 107, 110, 111, 116, 117-
      29, 131-33, 185, 203, 247
  auscultation of the lungs, 126, 167